STAYING HARD

The Only Exercise Book You Will Ever Need

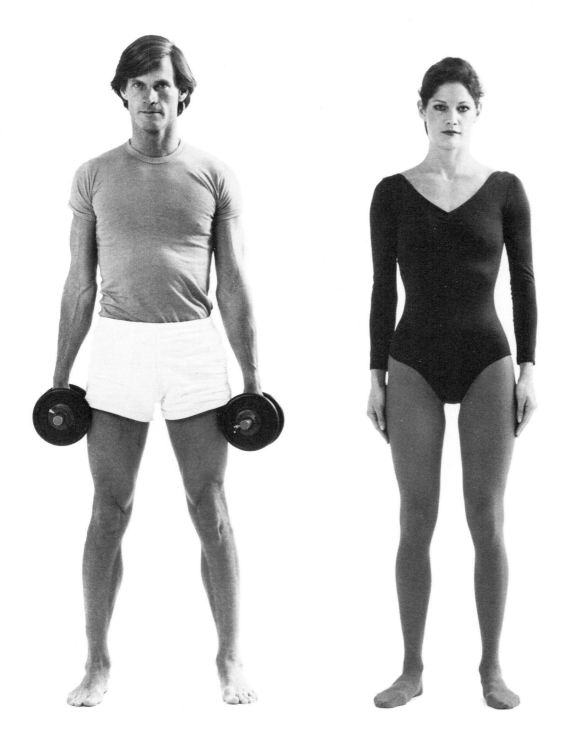

Also by Charles Gaines STAY HUNGRY • DANGLER   Also by Charles Gaines and George Butler PUMPING IRON

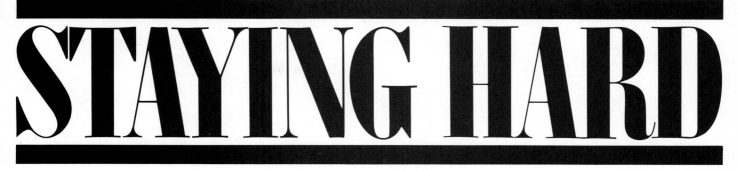

STAYING HARD

The Only Exercise Book You Will Ever Need

Written by Charles Gaines

Designed by Martin Stephen Moskof

Photographs of George Butler by Humphrey Sutton

All photographs taken in the Humphrey Sutton Studio in New York City

Kenan Press · New York

A Simon & Schuster Division of Gulf & Western Corporation
Simon & Schuster Building
Rockefeller Center
1230 Avenue of the Americas
New York, New York 10020
KENAN PRESS is a trademark of Simon & Schuster

Manufactured in the United States of America
Printed and bound by The Murray Printing Company
   3 4 5 6 7 8 9 10

Library of Congress Cataloging in Publication Data

Gaines, Charles, date.
  Staying hard.

  1. Exercise.   I. Butler, George, date.
II. Title.
GV461.G25   613.7   80-36698
ISBN 0-671-41265-5

Universal Gym Equipment courtesy of Universal Viking
Fitness Company, Plainview, Long Island, N.Y.
All other exercise equipment courtesy of
    Paragon Sporting Goods Company, Inc.,
    871 Broadway, New York City.

For Bob Dattila

True Hard

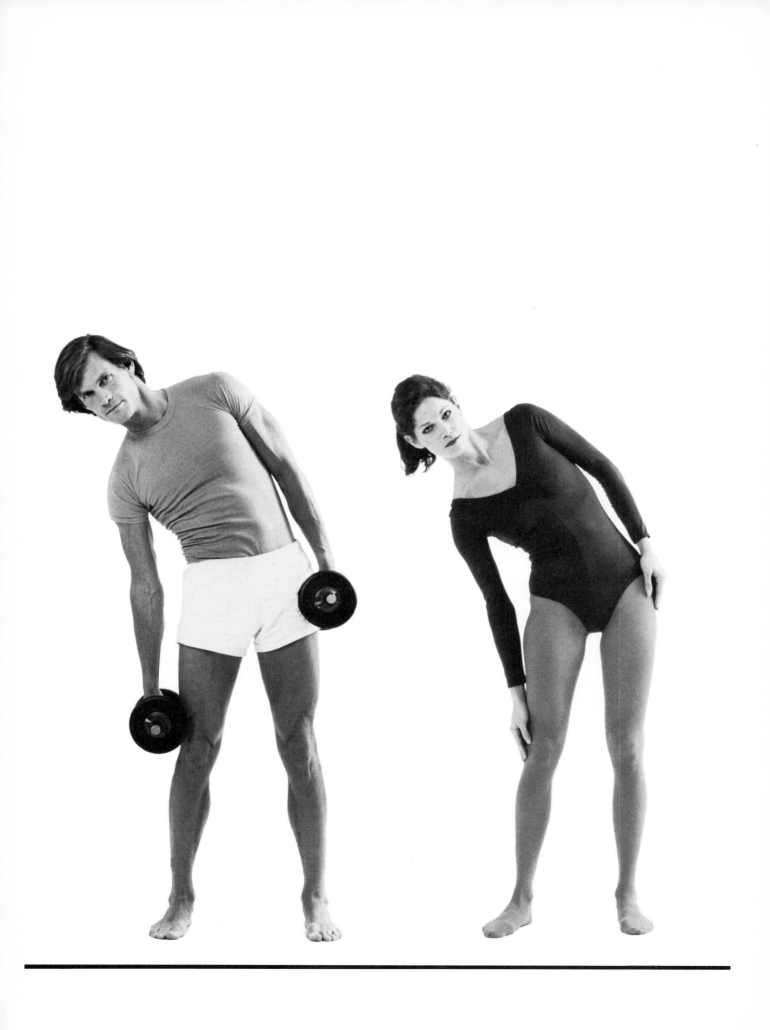

Contents

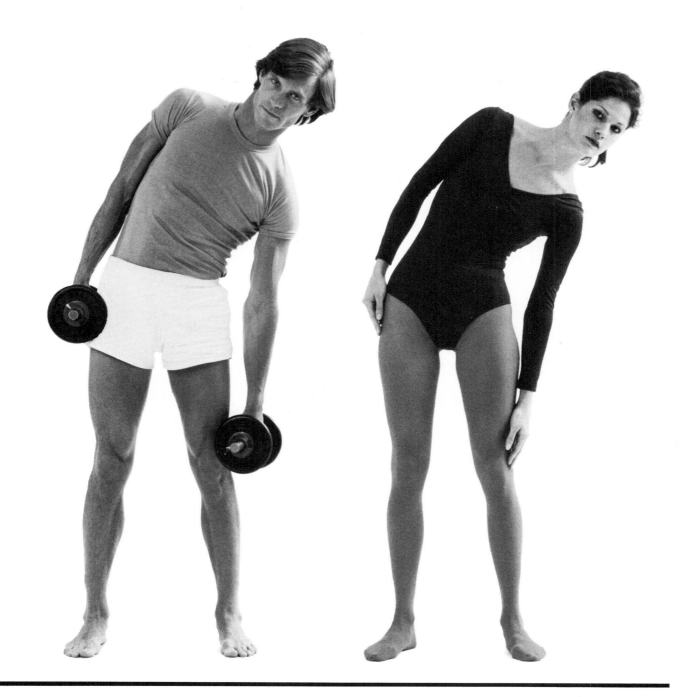

"In soft regions are born soft men (and women)."
—*Herodotus*

_____

"But they can be made hard."
—*Anonymous*

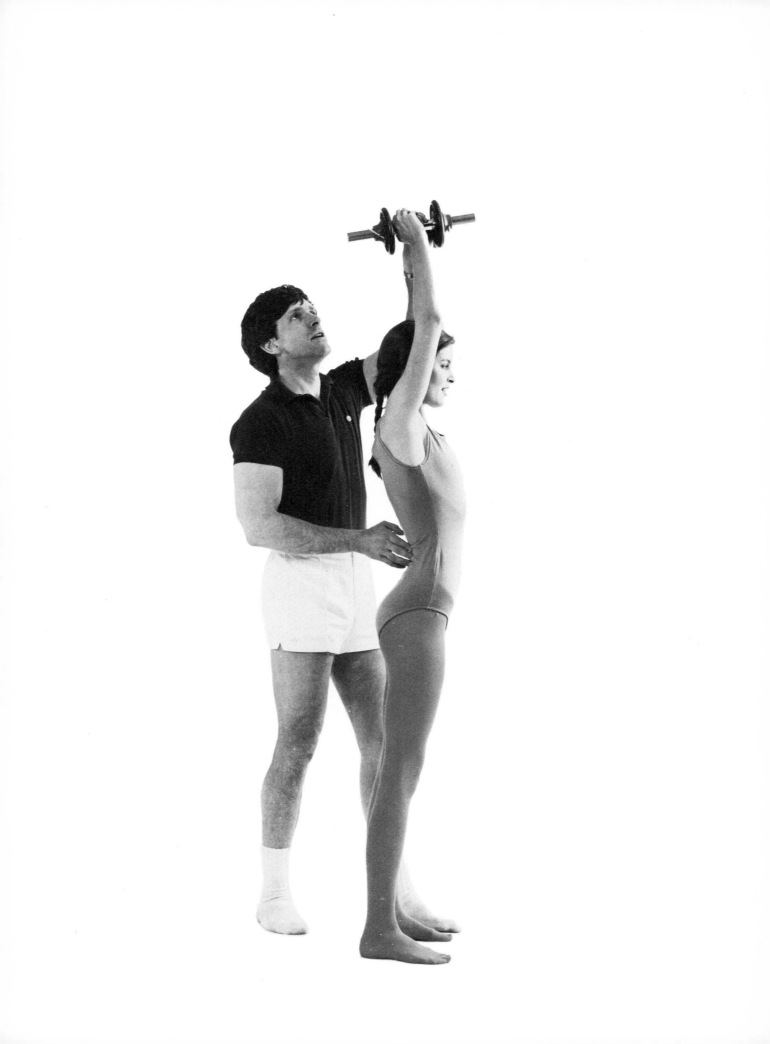

·I·
INTRODUCTION

A Note About the Author

I am thirty-seven years old and I sit at a desk to make my living. I smoke black cigars from Brazil, drink a lot of good whiskey, and eat whatever I want. Though I play at a lot of sports, I play at none of them with exceeding strenuousness or skill, and I insist on the option to overindulge—in work, sloth, food, drink, or sex—whenever I feel like it.

Despite all of the above, I am hard. I wake up hard every morning, go to bed hard every night. I enjoy that. If you are not hard, you probably remember what it felt like when you were and wish you were again; if you are, you undoubtedly enjoy it as I do and want to stay that way. In either case, man or woman, young or old, you need this book.

What Is "Hard"?

On the simplest level, the word "hard" here refers to the way your body feels to your own and other people's fingers. It doesn't mean hard like concrete—nobody wants to feel that way. It means pleasant hard; hard as opposed to doughy, and no one should want to feel doughy either. Our flesh is made up of fat and muscle tissue. Fat is mushy and yielding to the touch, and so is untoned muscle. Toned muscle (not at all the same as big muscle) is resilient and firm. It doesn't droop at the back of an arm, or sag at the bosom, or roll over a belt. On either a man or woman, toned muscle is much more fun to feel than fat or untoned muscle. It doesn't run in your hands; it springs back when you push it; it *responds* and has a feel to it of efficiency, for tone is to a body what sharpness is to a knife.

On the next level up in this context, "hard" refers to a particular kind of good physical shape, desirable for reasons I'm about to go into and achievable only by the kind of rigorous physical labor that nobody does anymore, or by the exercises in this book.

On its highest level, "hard" describes a way of living.

Why Stay Hard?

1. Because, male or female, you look better that way—in and out of clothes. And no matter what you may have heard, all of us want to look better.

2. Because, hard, you are just plain more enjoyable to touch, both for yourself and for other people.

3. Because you think, feel, and operate better hard than soft. A movie actress with the world's most perfect nose, once felt my leg and said: "Mmm. You don't get tired, do you?"

"Of course I get tired," I told her.

"Maybe you get *tired* tired. But not logy tired, I bet."

She was right. Hard, you rarely feel logy tired, potty, or stunned in the mind. You can withstand physical, emotional, and/or mental stress for longer periods than soft people, and you will find yourself generally more alert, more tolerant, and less nervous than they are. All of this is true. It is also true that, hard, you are less susceptible to injuries both physical and emotional.

4. Because being hard makes you feel better about overeating, overdrinking, staying up late at night, and other indulgences. Also, hard, you will recover from hangovers more quickly than soft people.

5. Because the conditioning exercises in this book that will make you or keep you hard will also make you or keep you better at sports and games than most people who are not hard. I say "most people" because all of us who are hard have at least one soft friend who can beat our socks off at various sports and games. I have a number of such friends, but that does not change the principle; and the fact is that to a man (or a woman) those friends will be ex-hard people, usually in an early stage of disintegration.

6. Because when you are hard you have a more satisfying sex life. You have a more satisfying sex life because, hard, you are better as both a lover and a lovee. In honesty, the same exceptions apply here as in number 5.

But Is This Really the Right Exercise Book For Me?

Yes. No matter who you are, if you are interested in staying or becoming hard, this is certainly the right exercise book for you.

But though the book can be used profitably by house-wives, children, old people—in fact, anyone who can read—it is directed at a sort of ideal, composite reader. That reader can every bit as well be a woman as a man. In the past ten years women's attitudes about exercise have changed right along with their attitudes about almost every-thing else. Mild cardiovascular exercise and languid stretch-ings are no longer enough for many, many women who have grown impatient with soft, flabby bodies and are willing to pull and push—to work, in a word—to avoid them. This book is perfect for such women, but for illustrative purposes, let's say that its ideal composite reader is a man. His name, let's say, is Phil, and he is thirty-three years old. He lives in a lovely house in Connecticut from which he commutes five days a week to his job in New York City.

Phil is an advertising executive and he earns over fifty thousand dollars a year. The pressures of his work are tre-mendous but he enjoys them. He enjoys the meetings and the travel and making up new campaigns. The work never seems to get old to him and he hopes that it never does, because Phil is an active and energetic person. At Yale, where he went to college, Phil played football, basketball, and tennis. Though he was not particularly outstanding at any of these sports he played them hard and competitively. Now he still plays tennis whenever he can, he skis ten or twelve times a winter, and he jogs two miles every Saturday and Sunday no matter what the weather.

Though he will still take a drink or two, Phil stopped smoking three years ago and he tries to eat carefully, even though he doesn't always do it. He cares about his body. He likes for it to look and feel good and he is proud of the things he can still do well with it. It is a good body, athletic, adaptable, and—up until recently—hard. Now, despite the jogging and the tennis, the skiing and all the skipped des-serts, it is going soft. Not fat, exactly, but soft. Phil can grab almost a handful of mush at either side of his waist. His chest is beginning to sag. He can feel his buttocks jiggle when he jogs, and the backs of his arms have gotten floppy.

Like a lot of you out there, Phil is losing his hard, and he doesn't want to. Staying hard is very important to him, because to him *being* hard is something more than just the tactile result of physical conditioning. He is still hard enough to know, or feel, that on its highest level of definition, "hard" is durability, discipline, energy, potency; it is more to bring to life and the readiness to bring it. It seems to Phil that for someone like himself—an affluent, sedentary American over college age—staying hard is having his cake and eating it too: the best possible revenge. It is outsmarting life, and he is determined to do it. Now with this book he can. And so can you, whoever you are.

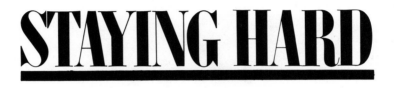

STAYING HARD

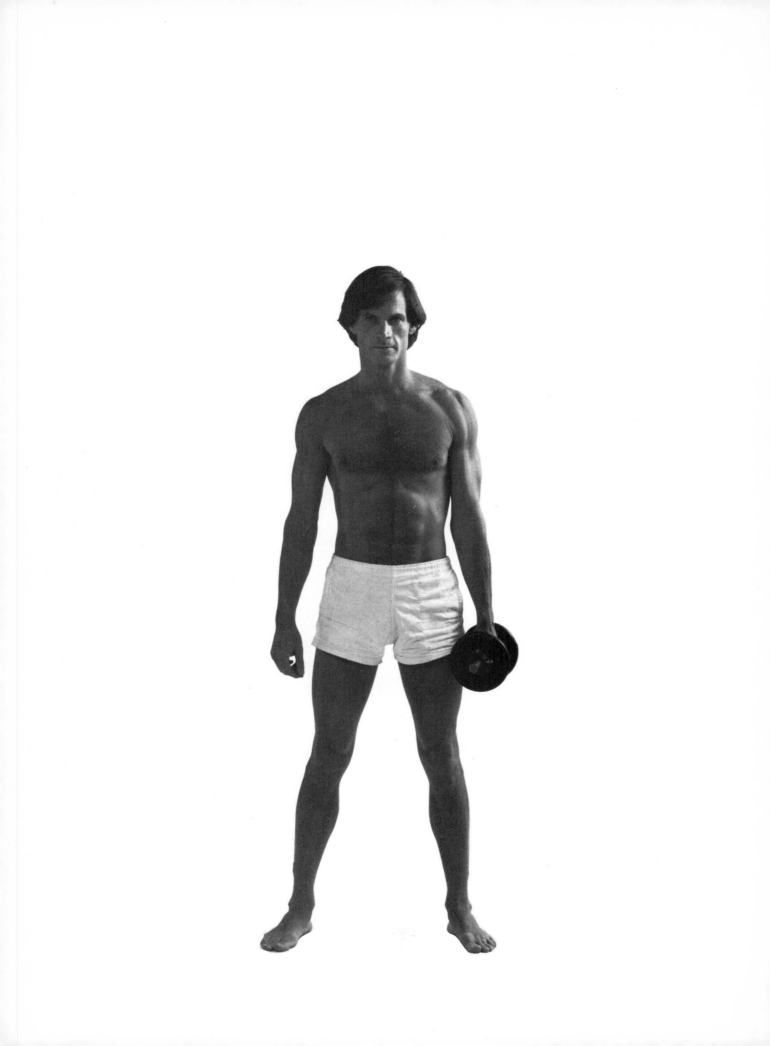

·II·
DOING IT

In the spring of 1978 the New Hampshire Bar Association, a jolly society of some six hundred lawyers, invited me up to their annual meeting at a big resort hotel in northern New Hampshire to discuss and demonstrate exercise.

"We don't want to look like your muscle-men buddies," said the lawyer who phoned me, referring to my previous journalistic association with competitive bodybuilders. "We just want to learn some kind of easy exercise routine that will keep us from going to pot."

"Soft," I corrected him. "Going soft."

"Whatever. It shouldn't take much time, though, and you should be able to do it anywhere. Can you come up with something like that?"

As it happened, I already had. A few years earlier I had spent some time in Birmingham, Alabama, working on the film of my first book, *Stay Hungry.* One of the stars of that film was my friend Arnold Schwarzenegger, at that time still Mr. Olympia and the top bodybuilder in the world. Arnold and I worked out together often in Birmingham at the downtown YMCA, and one afternoon a man came up and asked if either of us knew of a short, coherent program of muscle-toning exercises which could be done in a half hour or less, did not require weights, and could be performed in an office or a motel. The man said he was an executive with IBM; he traveled a lot and was not always near a gym. Neither Arnold nor I knew of such a program, though we could think of exercises that would be appropriate for it. We talked about it a little and I decided to try to come up with something, both for the IBM man and myself, for it occurred to me then that a program like the one he described—or better, a number of different programs—was exactly what I wanted as well.

At that point I had been lifting weights, seriously if never competitively, for twenty years. I love pumping iron, and wrote about how much I love it in a book of that name. I love the peculiar stress and energy of it, and how it makes your body feel, and I can't imagine a time when I would want to quit doing it entirely. But as you get older and

busier, particularly if you travel a lot, there are problems with strict weight training as your only, or even your major, method of staying hard. For one thing, conventional weight training is really more about *building* muscle than toning it, and few people over thirty are interested in having big muscles, including me. For another, you have to go someplace, usually a gym, to train with weights, and often there is no gym where you are, or, if there is, you don't have time to go to it. And for a third, unless you have your own gym or access to one at three o'clock in the morning, pumping iron is a social form of exercise, done amid a lot of groaning and heaving that is not your own. Though I used to enjoy that fact about it as much as any, more recently I have preferred as often as not to heave and groan alone.

I was ready—I learned from the IBM man in Birmingham —for a Dopp-Kit exercise program: something light, accessible, portable, and personal, that I could take with me wherever I went. And when, three years later, the lawyer in New Hampshire called me, I had it—not just one but a number of them, each with its own personality, each a compatible assortment of exercises invented or adapted to meet particular circumstances in a lot of different places around the world.

I had the programs, but up until the day I demonstrated them to the New Hampshire Bar Association they were my own private Dopp-Kits—full of used, personal things, well traveled but private. Since then I've showed them, or parts of them, to quite a few other people, most recently to a big, yellow-haired German model on a barge in the Hudson River who, ignoring the party we were there for, got down on the floor in her velvet pants and heaved and groaned magnificently for over an hour learning them. In showing them around I've had to adjust them, take out something here, put in something there, to accommodate different individuals and purposes—and now they are no longer private. In fact they are now so public that anyone can do them, I hope with as much appetite and purpose as that German model. And that's the reason for this book.

In addition to the free-exercise programs, included here are three programs I developed to be done in the home or office using only two small dumbbells and a barbell, and three more designed for the growing number of people who own or have easy access to a Universal machine. But before I get into how you are supposed to use all these specific exercise programs, a few words about exercise in general.

Distinguished by their primary effects on the body, there are three broad categories of exercises: cardiovascular, stretching, and resistant. Though there is always some overlap, and often quite a bit, each of the three categories is aimed at achieving a separate set of results. Put simply (there is absolutely no need to put it more complexly) the primary effect of training by means of cardiovascular exercises such as running or swimming is to condition the lungs and heart. The primary effect of stretching exercises is to lengthen and make more flexible the muscles and tendons, while that of resistant exercises is to build, strengthen, and tone them. First-rate overall fitness is an effect achieved only by a comprehensive daily training program that utilizes all three categories. Very few of us have time in our lives for that sort of training, so what most of us wind up doing with the time we do have for exercise is cheating in one direction or another. I have a yoga friend who is as flexible as a rubber doll but cannot chin himself. I know any number of guys with eighteen-inch arms who can't run a mile, and almost as many who can and do run five miles a day but whose waists or backs or chests are flabby and soft.

Let me say this now: You cannot get *really* fit—I mean first-rate, world-class, decathlon fit—by using this book; nor can you by using any exercise book that I've ever seen. You have to devote most of your life to exercise to get that kind of fit, and no book could tell you how to do it even if there were one that tried. The programs in *Staying Hard* are made up mostly of resistant exercises, because resistance is what makes and keeps you hard. But there are enough stretching exercises in each program to keep you as flexible as most of us need to be, and by completing each program within or near its Target Time you will derive some cardiovascular benefit as well. Not very much, to be honest. Ideally, you should supplement the exercises here with running or swimming if you are interested in excellent cardiovascular fitness.

Now, having disclaimed, let me claim: If what you are interested in doing is getting or staying hard, the programs in this book are all you will ever need; if what you want is to get in and stay in as good overall shape as possible with a limited amount of time to devote to exercise, then all you will ever need are the programs in this book plus an equal amount of running or swimming time (e.g., half an hour a day, three days a week, to a program; half an hour a day, three days a week, to running or swimming).

Remember, before starting any exercise program, it is always advisable to consult a doctor.

Not only does this book offer you all you will ever need to stay hard and fit, but it will accommodate anyone, either sex, any age. And not only that, but it doesn't matter where you are starting from: Someone just out of a hospital can do the exercises in Program One; Bruce Jenner could get sore on Programs Six or Nine.

The exercises are divided into three sections, and there are three programs (beginner, intermediate, and advanced) in each section. The sections themselves are not arranged progressively; that is to say, Program Five, which is in the second section, is no harder or easier than Program Two, which is in the first, or Program Eight, which is in the third—just different. You can stay hard by doing only the programs in one section, though personally I like to mix them. When I'm traveling I do exercises from Section I; when I'm at home or at my office and don't have time to go to a gym, I do routines similar to the ones in Section II; and I do exercises from Section III whenever I have access to a Universal machine.

Here is how to determine where you should start within any of the three sections:

Pick the section that appeals to you most or best fits your life. Do the first program of the section. Do each exercise exactly as instructed. If you cannot complete the entire program in (or within a few seconds of) its Target Time, without giving yourself a heart attack or getting sore as hell the next day, stick with it until you can. If you can do the first program within its Target Time, test yourself in the same way on the next. If you fail, that's where you should start. If you pass, go on to the advanced program of the section.

If you can do any of the advanced programs the first time within its Target Time and without soreness or exhaustion, I need to be reading your book.

After you have determined where to begin, do so. At once. And then keep at it. Do the program three days a week (four or five if you can), trying to speed up a little each time. When you get within a few seconds of the Target Time, go on to the next program. After you have gotten to where you can consistently complete the advanced program within its Target Time, you can add sets or repititions if you want to, or more weight in the case of Programs Six and Nine. Or you can go on to another section.

But there is no need to do any of that. Any of the advanced programs, as is, done three to five days a week, will keep you exactly the right degree of hard for as long as you continue to do it.

At the back of this book, along with a few idiosyncratic diet tips, is a chart naming the major muscles you will be concerned with and telling you where they are located. There are over six hundred muscles in the human body. Many of them operate involuntarily. Others, like the muscles around the face and in the hands and forearms, are used voluntarily so often that toning them is unnecessary. For the purposes of *Staying Hard,* the rest of the voluntary muscles can be divided into six groups, or areas of the body: the waist, the legs and buttocks, the chest, the back, the shoulders, and the arms. It is the major muscles of these groups that are listed and located for reference in the back.

For a couple of reasons the muscle groups should be exercised in the sequence they are listed above: First, because in any general routine large muscles should always be worked before the smaller supporting ones; second, because the area-by-area progression of the body toward soft usually follows the same sequence, and you want to hit your most vulnerable areas while you are freshest.

There are two terms that should be defined before we get into how to do the exercises—terms that quantify them. A *rep,* or repetition, is one full performance of the exercise; a *set* is a given number of repetitions done consecutively. While the prescribed number of sets per exercise in each of these programs is never more than one, the number of repetitions per set is relatively high. I have found that for toning, as opposed to building, muscles—for staying hard—more than one set of an exercise is unnecessary if there are sufficient repetitions in the set to "burn" the muscle. In building muscles the physical effect you are after, following a given exercise, is a "pump"—the oxygenated swell of torn-down muscle tissue that is requisite to growth. In toning, what you want after each set is a burning sensation in the worked area, which lets you know you have reached and tired the major muscles there without breaking them down. A pump means growth; a burn means tone.

Also, the repetitions in these routines, except where noted otherwise, should be done as quickly as you can do them in good form, and you should wait as little time as possible between exercises: not longer than a minute, and ideally as few as ten to fifteen seconds. The word "burn" has a second application here: A lot of repetitions done quickly like this not only tone and harden muscles but help burn off the adipose tissue surrounding them.

All right, so you have picked the section of exercises that best suits you, and have tested yourself to determine which of its programs you should start with. You know to do the repetitions quickly, and to rest as little time as possible between exercises. What else?

A number of things:

1. *Do it at a regular time.* Pick a time of the day to do the exercises and try to stick with it, even when you are traveling. Exercise is a habit, and like any habit it thrives on schedule. Since none of the programs should require more than forty or forty-five minutes to complete, and most of them less than thirty, any daily routine no matter how busy should be able to accommodate a program at a particular time of day or night. I like to do it first thing in the morning —to get hard for my day before I really begin it. But any time (except for right after a meal) is OK, and some have specific virtues. If you tend to overeat in the middle of the day, try doing the program right before lunch and watch how it cuts your appetite. If you're trying to cut down on your drinking before dinner, schedule your program where the shank of your drinking time used to be. If you have trouble sleeping at night, do the program an hour before you go to bed.

The important thing is that you stick to the schedule. If four to four-thirty in the afternoon is your time for doing it, do it then, no matter what. If four to four-thirty is often impossible for you, pick another time.

2. *Do it without missing.* There are thousands, maybe millions, of soft people out there who say, "Who, me? Of course I exercise. I'm just soft because my momma was soft —it's in my genes." Something like that. The truth could be that they exercise improperly, or lazily, or too little. But chances are the truth is this: They do it *every once in a while.*

Doing it every once in a while just won't get it. Not much is being asked here—approximately a half hour to forty-five minutes a day, three days a week. For that you want hard and you get hard; for any less, you don't. There hasn't been a single day in years that I have missed doing some program of exercise, sick or well, no matter how busy I was. There's no need for you to be that obsessive about not missing— just committed to it.

3. *Do it with concentration.* In this life, you can't even drink a beer well if you don't concentrate on it. Don't ask me why—it's just a fact. So is this: If you don't put your head in these exercises you won't stay hard on them. They were developed with concentration (mine), and they have to be performed with it (yours).

But maybe you don't know what it means to concentrate on exercise. What it means first is coming to that time three days a week you have chosen to do it with your mind more or less clear of all the stuff that clutters it up at other times. Then it means keeping your attention on the exercises while you do them; and finally it means thinking through each exercise individually—burying your head in each repetition, thinking the muscles through it. Basically it's the same as concentrating on anything else—it means giving yourself over to it.

Throughout the programs, you will be urged to "feel" certain exercises. This is a function of concentration, and it is not difficult to do, no matter how new you are to exercise. Just be aware of the movements you are making, locate in your mind the muscular sensation, or *feel*, produced by them, and then concentrate on that feel through each repetition.

4. *Do it according to an image of yourself.* Before you start the program, take off your clothes and look at yourself in a full-length mirror. Look honestly. If you are perfectly happy with what you see, fine; the programs in the book will keep you happy. If you see areas that bother you, feel them. More than likely they are soft. Now imagine yourself hard there: Get a visual and tactile image in your mind of how you want to look and feel, and think yourself toward that image while you are doing the exercises. Try to look in a mirror every time you finish your program. This is not narcissism; it is confrontation. If you want to stay hard, you have to confront your soft. Look at it, feel it, acknowledge it, and visualize it hard. Before long it will be.

Now you are ready, so go do it. Do it three days a week without missing, at a particular time, no matter where you are; do it with concentration and toward an improved visualization of yourself. Do it with joy, and tell your friends to do it.

Tell them this, as I'm telling you: "If you are going to stay at all, hard is the only way to do it."

·III·
THE EXERCISES

Section I:
Free Exercises

These are exercises that can be done almost anywhere and with a minimum of props. The few props that are required, I've learned, are easily found, borrowed, or stolen anywhere in the world. If you travel a lot, or dislike weights and machines, if you are attracted as I am by the notion of carrying your hard with you and being dependent on practically nothing for it, this is the section for you.

I didn't invent all the exercises here, but I did put them together, and the way they are put together is what is unique and significant about them. Because of the way they are put together, each program here and in the other two sections is more than just the sum of its parts. You could say that each program is like a different recipe for cooking pheasant: Some are easier than others; each has its own character; all of them work. All of them too have been considerably tested and refined, and for that reason you would probably do well to do them according to the recipes, at least until you are experienced enough to know what to add and what to leave out.

Here, as with all the programs, it is centrally important to do each exercise in good form. Try to do each repetition perfectly, concentrating on reaching the muscle as you do it. A major part of doing any exercise in good form is your breathing. You should always exhale on the resistance phase of the movement, and inhale on the relaxation phase. In a push-up, for example, inhale as your body is going down, exhale as it is going up.

These programs were designed so that they could be done as easily outside as indoors. Do them outside whenever you can—the fresh air will give you more energy. And do them in loose, moisture-absorbing clothes, if you have to do them in clothes at all.

One more thing: There is no need to warm up before starting any of the programs—a warm-up is built into each of them.

Program One

(Beginner)
Target Time:
Seventeen minutes

Waist

1. Bent-Leg Sit-Up:
One set.
Fifteen repetitions.

This is the easiest form of the best sit-up there is, bar none—the one favored by world-class bodybuilders. The function of this sit-up is to trim and tone the waist, not to strengthen it, and it works primarily on the upper abdominal and intercostal muscles.

Sitting up on the floor with your knees bent, place your feet under some stationary object. Clasp your hands together on your chest, keeping your elbows near your body. Holding your back straight, lower your upper body halfway to the floor and sit back up for one repetition. At the top of each repetition, tense your stomach muscles. Do the repetitions as fast as you can in good form.

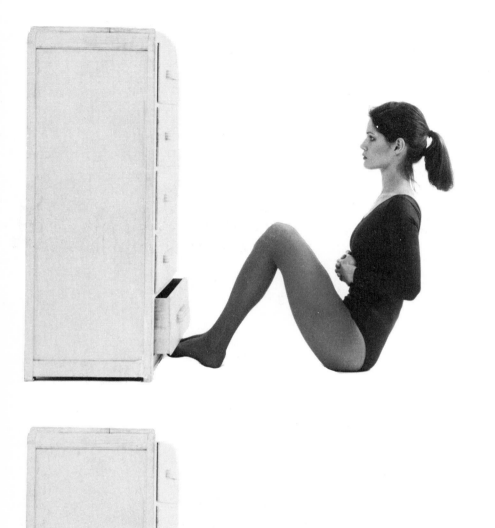

Waist

2. Knee-ups:
One set.
Fifteen repetitions.

This exercise is primarily for the lower abdominals, though it also exercises and massages the lower back and is good for people with problems there.

Lying flat on your back, your arms beside your body, bring your knees together into your chest. Then straighten your legs slowly and drop them to the floor for one repetition. Try to *feel* the lower abdominal muscles stretching as you straighten your legs.

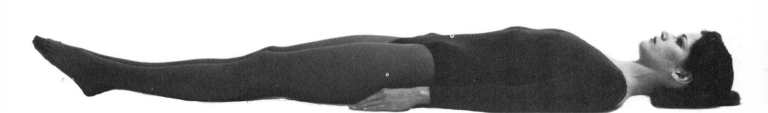

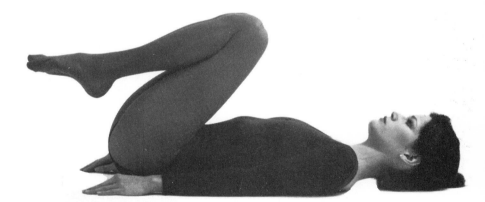

Waist

3. Side Bends:
One set.
Fifteen repetitions to each side.

Side bends tone the obliques, the muscles underneath the often-soft spots known as love handles. They too can be helpful to lower-back problems.

To do them, stand with your feet about twelve inches apart, your arms hanging at your sides. Bend sideways at the waist to the right, dropping your right hand as close as you can to the side of your right knee, then *lift* your body vertical again, using the obliques at the left side of your waist, which you should feel pulling as you come up. Now do the same thing on the other side.

Like many others here, this is a *feel* exercise: To get the most out of it you have to feel it in the area being toned, and to feel it you have to do the exercise correctly and concentrate.

Waist

4. Standing Twists:

One set.
Fifteen repetitions.

This one is good for all the abdominal muscles and is a fine flexibility exercise as well.

Stand with your feet shoulder-width apart, arms held out to sides at shoulder height. Keeping your arms straight and your hips facing forward, swing as far as you can to the right, then back through the vertical to the left for one repetition. Keep your feet flat on the floor.

Again, try to feel the exercise in your waist as you do it.

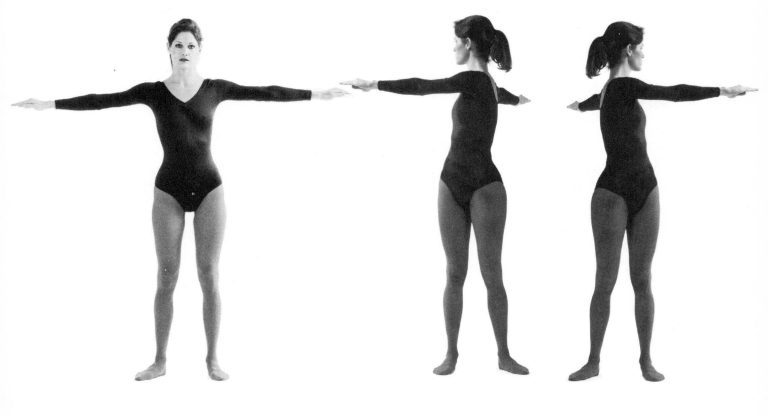

Legs and Buttocks

5. Aided Knee Bends to Chair:
One set.
Fifteen repetitions.

An easier version of the deep knee bend, this is a wonderful toning exercise for the upper legs (quadriceps) and buttocks. It is a very good exercise for downhill and cross-country skiing.

Stand with your feet shoulder width apart in front of something you can hold onto with your hands at waist to chest height, and with a chair beneath you. Keeping your back straight, lower your seat to the chair, then stand back up without lurching, letting the muscles of your frontal thighs lift you.

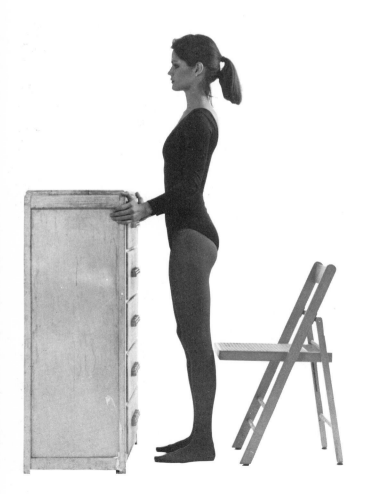
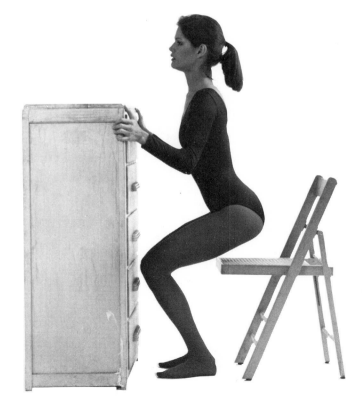

Legs and Buttocks

6. Isometric Leg Curls:
One Set.
Three repetitions with each leg.

Isometric exercises are ones in which resistance is created by tension against a fixed object. They really work, but in order for them to work well you have to feel them—in this case at the backs of the thighs, in the biceps femoris or hamstring muscles.

Bend over at the waist and hold onto something. Behind you there should be a table or an open drawer, or a diving board—anything that won't move—at about knee-joint height. Hook your right heel under it and pull upward and forward as if you were trying to bring the object to you. Get to full flexion of the muscle and hold it for five seconds. Then do the other leg. Alternate for three five-second repetitions with each leg.

Legs and Buttocks

7. Lying Side Leg Raises:
One set.
Fifteen repetitions with each leg.

This exercise is for hardening the buttocks and the sides of the thighs. It is also good for flexibility and is a good skiing and jogging conditioner.

Lie on your left side with your left arm supporting your head and your right hand on the floor or ground near your chest for balance. Keeping your right leg straight, raise it as high as you can and lower it again—quickly—for one repetition with that leg. When you have done fifteen, turn over and do the left leg. Feel it in the buttocks and along the sides of the thighs.

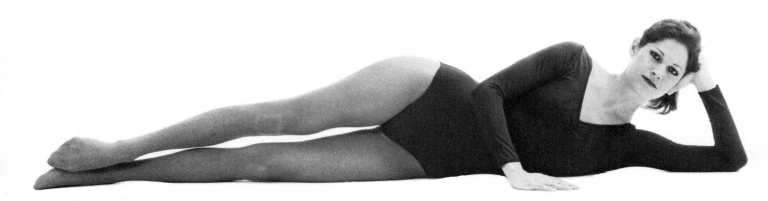

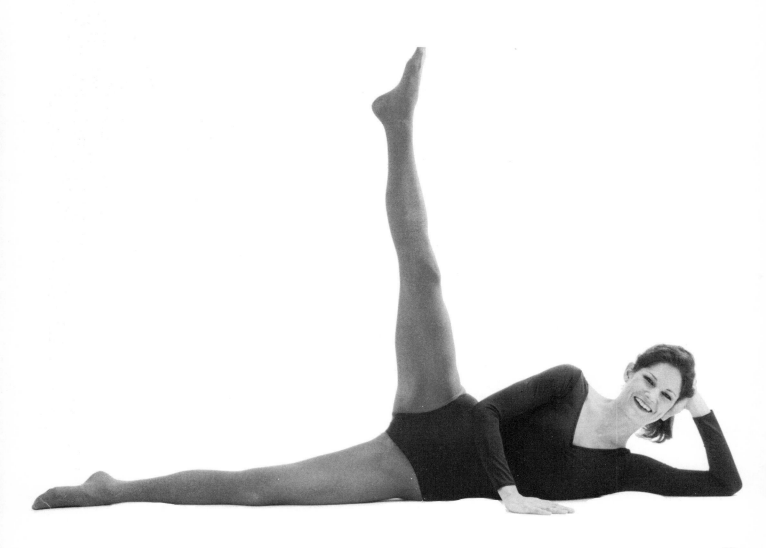

Legs and Buttocks

8. Two-Leg Calf Raises:
One set.
Fifteen repetitions.

Calves usually need less toning than other areas of the legs and buttocks but they often need shaping, and if you ski or bicycle or play basketball or skate, your calves can't be too hard. There are many variations of the calf raise, or toe stand; this is one of the easiest.

Find a large book, or rock, or some kind of ledge like the lip of a swimming pool, to stand on. Stand on it only with the balls of your feet and the first couple of inches of your instep, letting your heels hang off the back. Start with your heels dropped down as far as they will go, putting strain on the calf muscles, and stand up on the balls of your feet. Hold your peak position for a second or two, feeling the exercise in your calves, for one complete repetition.

Unlike most of the exercises here, this one should be done slowly.

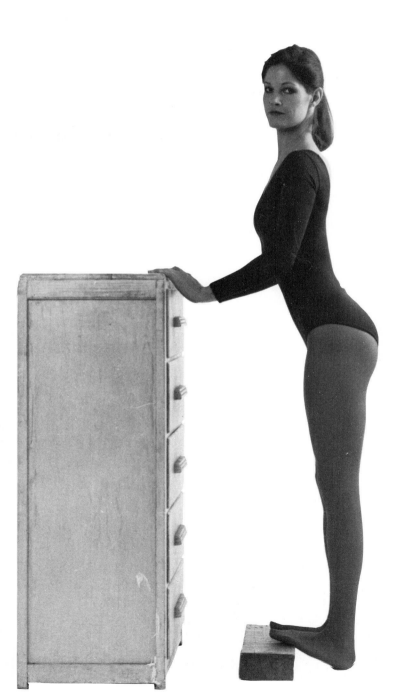
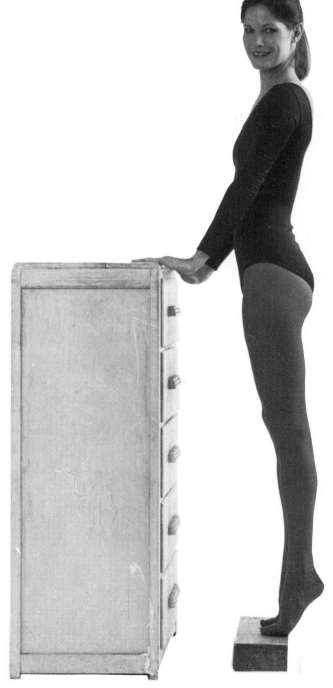

Chest

9. Push-ups Off Table:
One set.
Fifteen repetitions.

After the waist and upper legs, the chest, both male and female, is likely the next area to go soft on you. For some reason that I don't have, it also seems to be the area of the body that responds quickest to well-designed toning exercises—like this and the one that follows it.

This is an easy form of push-up. To do it, find a table, bench, dresser, rock wall—something about half your height. Stand in front of it, with your feet three feet away and a foot apart. Put your hands on the table, bench, etc., spacing them just outside your shoulders. Holding your back straight, lower yourself so that your chest touches the object (lower; don't drop to it), and then push back up until your arms are straight for one repetition.

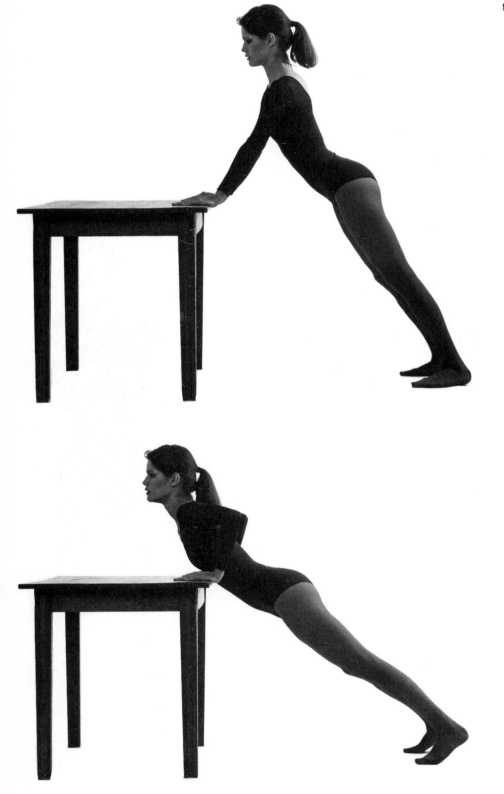

Chest

10. Standing Cross-Arm Flies:
One set.
Fifteen repetitions.

Push-ups work mostly on the center of the pectorals. Flies tone the outside wings of the muscles which run in to the frontal deltoids.

For this exercise, stand with your feet a couple of feet apart and your arms held straight out at your sides. Slowly, feeling it in the chest, cross your arms, left over right—pulling each across your chest as far as it will go—then bring them back to the original position for one rep. On the next rep, cross your right arm over your left, and continue to alternate through the set.

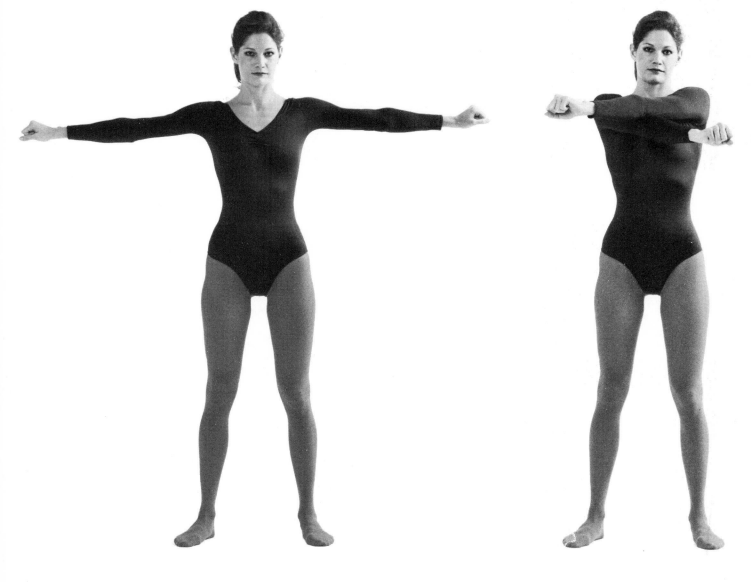

Back

11. Lying Lower-Back Extensions:
One set.
Fifteen repetitions.

The soft around the lower back ties in ominously with the soft around the waist. This exercise gets to it. It is an excellent flexibility exercise, good for lower-back problems, and wonderful for all sports, particularly tennis.

Lie down facing the ground or floor, your hands by your shoulders, palms down. Now lift up at the waist, helping as little as possible with your hands, until your chest and stomach, down to below your navel, are off the ground. Look up at the ceiling and hold the arch in your lower back for a second or two on each repetition.

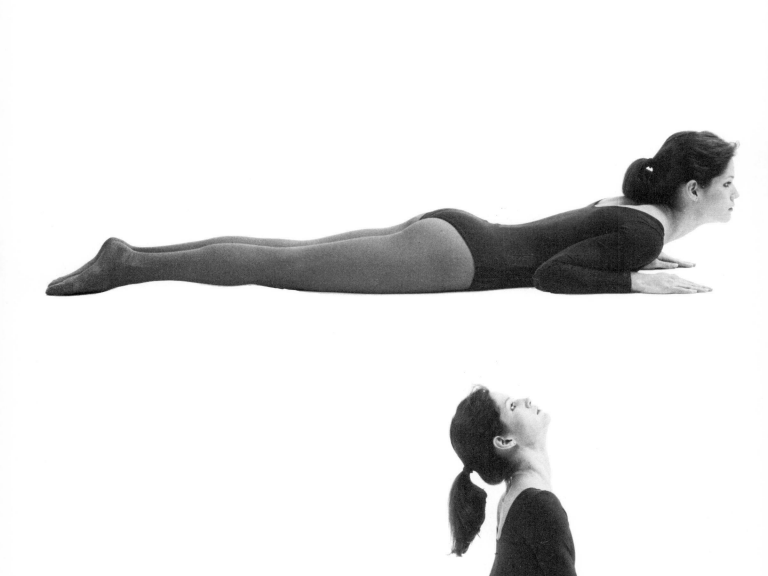

Back

12. Lat Pulls:
One set.
Fifteen repetitions.

The name of this exercise comes from the abbreviated name of the muscle it works—the latissimus dorsi. If you have any doubt as to whether this large back muscle goes soft, just go watch any noon YMCA basketball game among men over thirty and note the percentage of jiggling upper backs.

Stand in front of something solid which you can grip at chest height. Keep your feet wide and ten to twelve inches away from the object. Grab the object with both hands, lean back so that your arms are fully extended, and pull yourself to it, touching your chest. The pull should come from your back, not your arms. This is hard to describe, but easy to feel. If your arms are tired after the set you are doing it wrong: Next time make the pull come from the sides of your upper back.

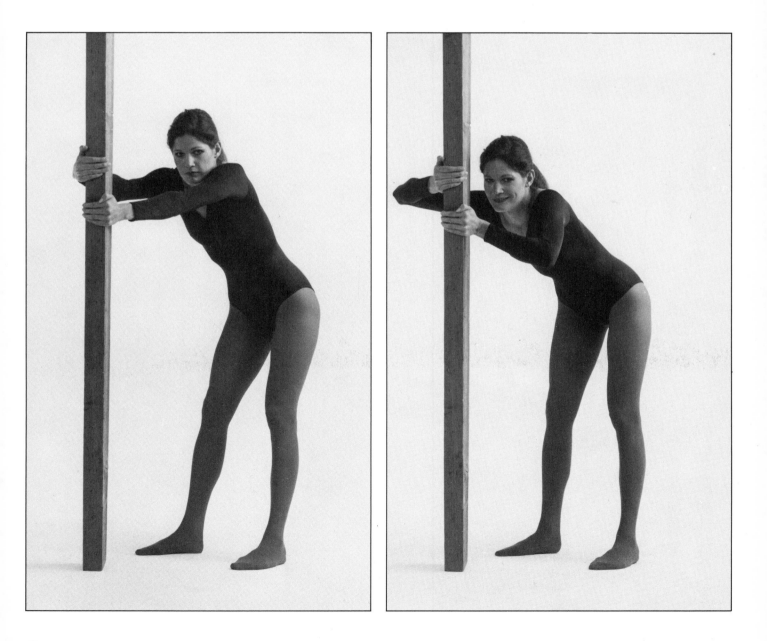

Shoulders

13. Push-offs:
One set.
Fifteen repetitions.

This and the next exercise tone the deltoid or shoulder muscles. They are good conditioning exercises for any racquet sport, volleyball, basketball, and, particularly, cross-country skiing.

To do the push-offs, you'll need another table, bench, chair, etc., something less than waist height. Standing with feet two to three feet apart and three feet from the object, place your hands on the object, spacing them a little wider than your shoulders. Now bend at the waist so that your back goes flat and on a plane with your hands. Let your head come in to touch the table or whatever, and then push off from it, keeping your back level. Here again, if you are doing the exercise correctly, you will feel it in your shoulders.

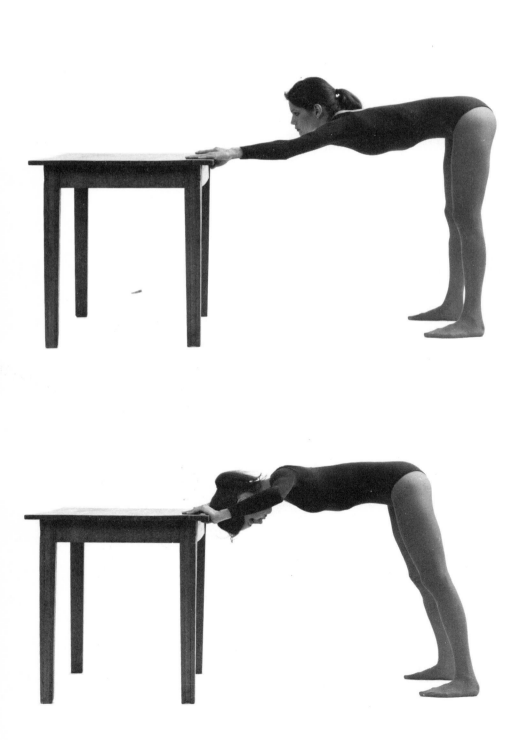

Shoulders

14. Standing Front and Lateral Flies:
One set.
Ten repetitions.

This exercise has the same athletic benefits as the previous one, and works both the frontal and rear deltoids. You will need more than the usual concentration to do it correctly.

Stand with your back straight, your fists clenched, and your arms bowed a little at your sides. Now raise both arms straight in front of you to chest level, imagining—feeling—them weighted; then lower them and raise them in the same way to ear level out to your sides for one full repetition. Do ten repetitions, and throughout each make your arms struggle to rise.

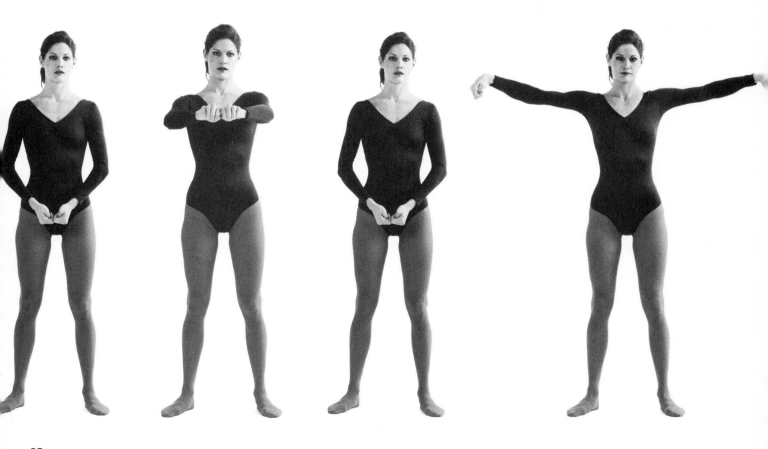

Arms

15. Standing Curls:
One set.
Fifteen repetitions with each arm.

The muscles at the front and back of the upper arms go soft very quickly when not used, and not many of us use them in everyday life. They are important muscles to swimming, rowing and paddling, tennis, climbing, and many other sports—and they feel very good to the touch when they are toned, and lousy when they are not.

This first exercise is for the biceps. To do it you will need a couple of large books, or other objects of similar weight.

Stand with your feet together, arms at your side, holding the books with your palms facing upward. Keeping your back and upper arm straight (the elbow should not lift up), curl the book in your right hand up to shoulder height and lower it again for a repetition. Alternate arms for fifteen reps apiece.

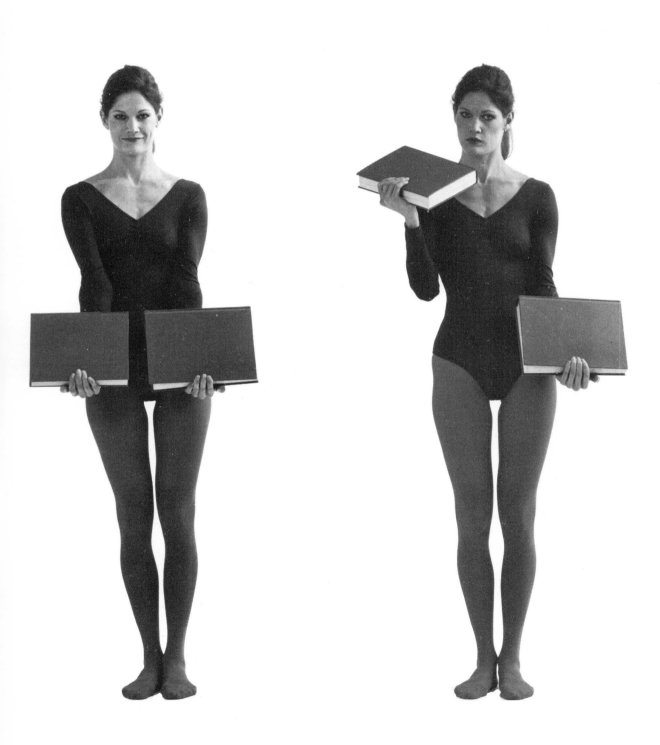

Arms

16. Triceps Push-offs:
One set.
Fifteen repetitions.

For those saggy backs of upper arms you see, and feel, more and more now.

Again, stand in front of something about the height of a table or a desk, with your feet about three feet away from it and shoulder width apart. Put the heels of your palms on the object, with only a few inches between your hands. Now, using your elbows as hinges, drop your head to your hands and push back up for one repetition.

This exercise might take some getting used to before you can isolate the movement in the triceps. If you're doing it correctly you should feel it only in the backs of your arms and not in your shoulders.

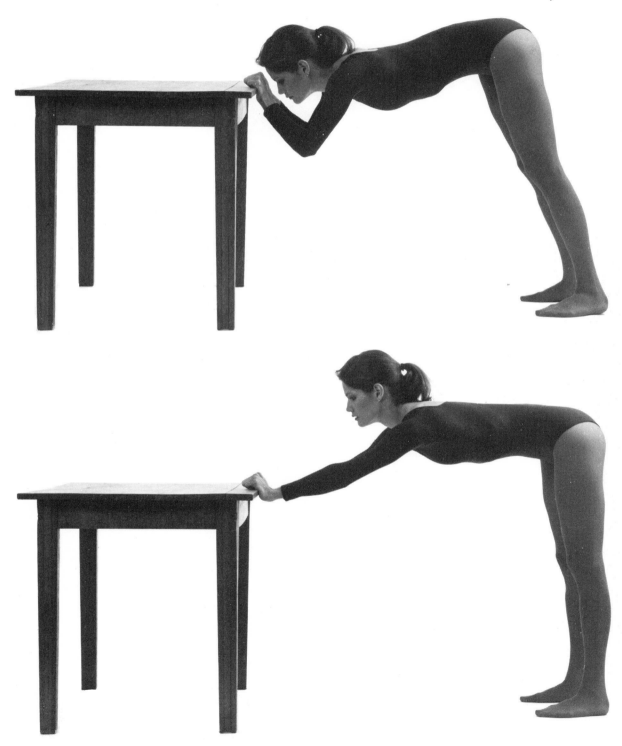

Program Two

(Intermediate)
Target Time:
Twenty-two minutes

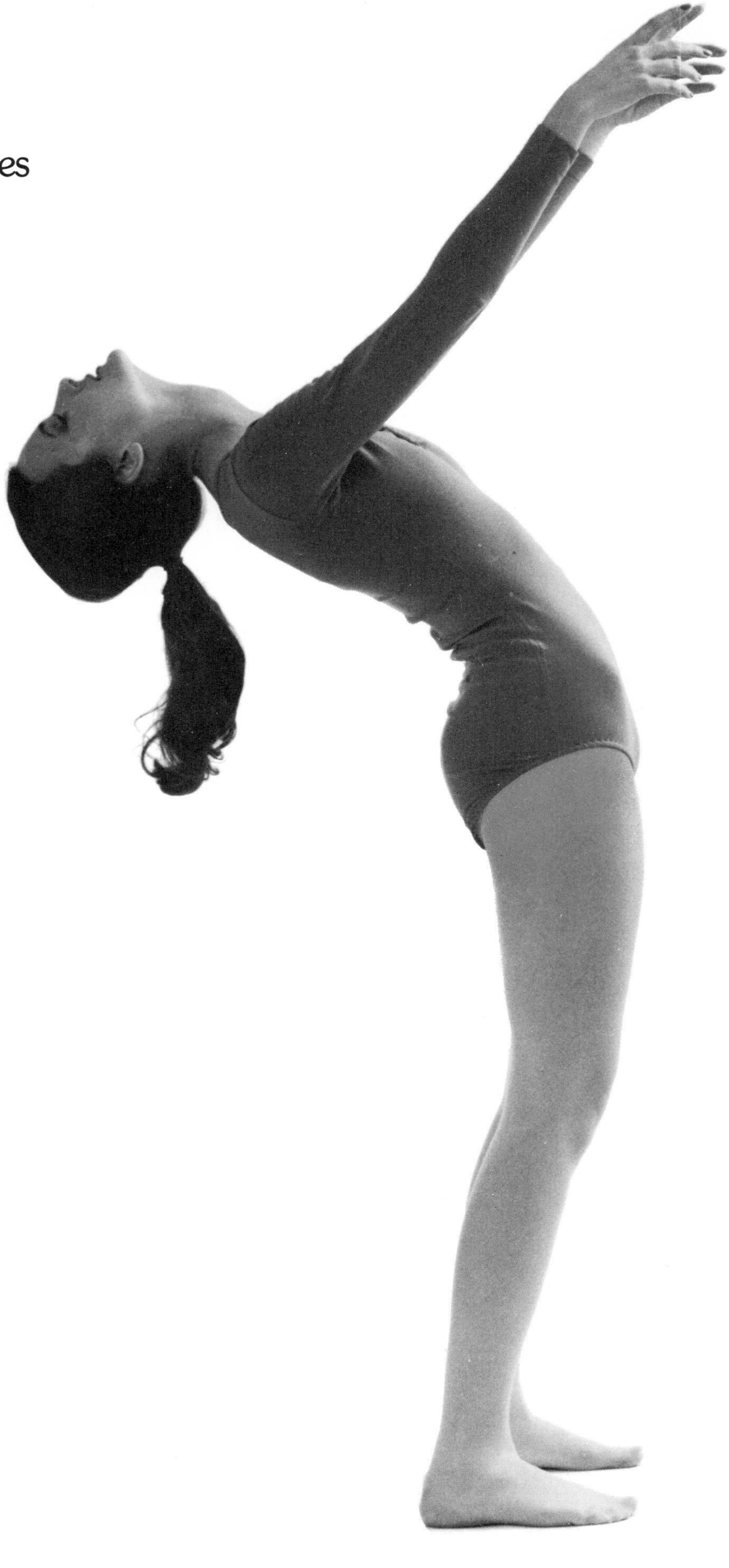

Waist

17. Bent-Leg Sit-ups:
One set.
Fifty repetitions.

This is a somewhat more difficult version of the sit-up in Program One (Exercise 1). Sit on the floor with your knees bent and your feet under something stationary. Holding your arms by your side, drop back far enough so that your lower back touches the floor before sitting up for one repetition. Do them fast. You should feel them in your upper abdominals.

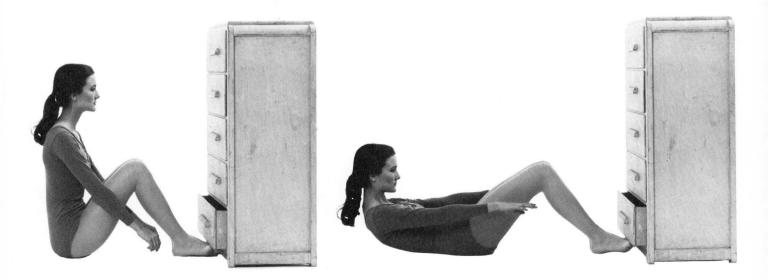

Waist

18. Leg Raises:
One set.
Twenty repetitions.

Like the knee-ups in Program One, this exercise hardens the lower abdominals and is good for the lower back.

With your arms spread wide on the floor, raise your legs to vertical. Raise them, don't heave them up; and lower, rather than drop, them to the floor on the way down.

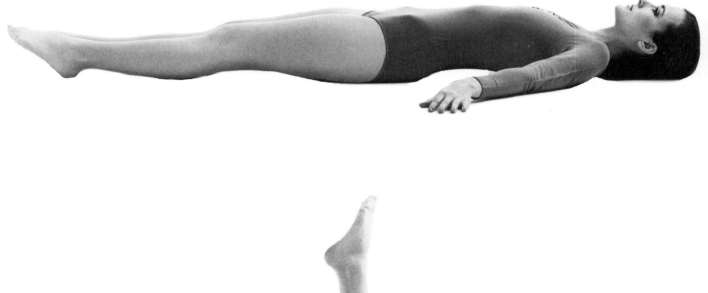

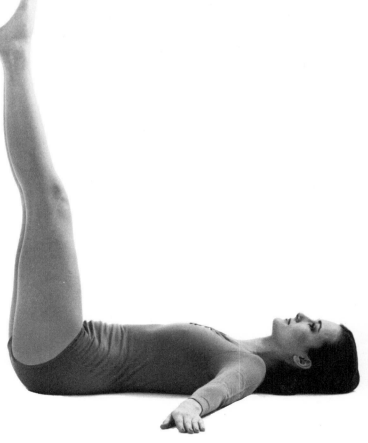

Waist

19. Side Bends:
One set.
Twenty repetitions to each side.

To harden the oblique muscles at the sides of your waist.

Stand with your feet a comfortable distance apart. Keeping your back straight, drop your right arm so that your right hand comes level with your knee, at the same time swinging your left arm up to where it is pointed at the ceiling—feel the stretch along your left side. Do this twenty times. Then do twenty to the other side, dropping your left arm and swinging up your right.

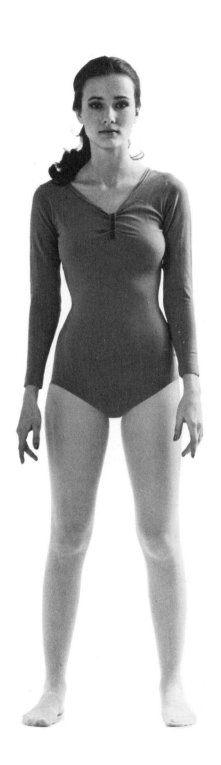

Waist

20. Seated Twists:
One set.
Twenty repetitions to each side.

This works on all the major abdominal muscles and is very good for torso flexibility.

Sit in a chair and extend your arms out to the side. Keep your arms straight and twist at the waist as far as you can around to the right for one repetition, then back around to the left for one on that side.

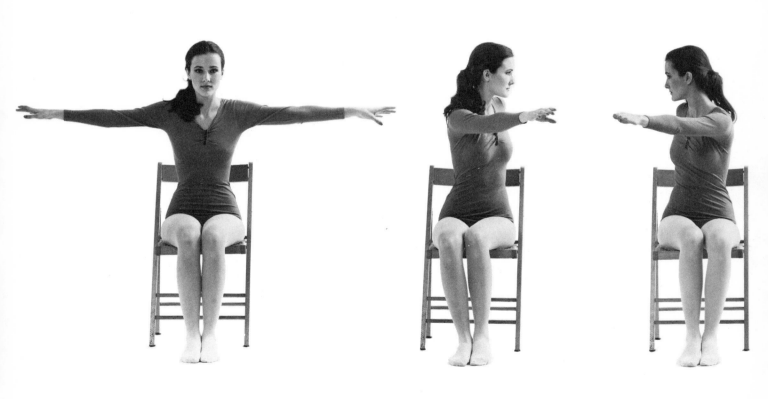

Waist

21. Back Bends:
One set.
Ten repetitions.

Though this exercise also strengthens and tones the lower back, when done correctly it is a wonderful toner for the frontal waist muscles.

From a standing position, bend backward as far as you can, letting your arms ride up in front of your chest. Now, using your abdominal muscles, pull (don't jerk) yourself upright.

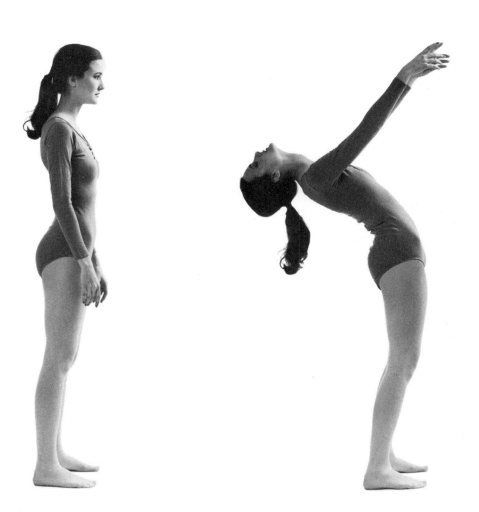

An excellent exercise for all sports.

22. Deep Knee Bends:
One set.
Twenty repetitions.

Hold onto something below waist height for balance if necessary, but don't use it to pull up on. Your feet should be about six inches apart. Keep your back straight going down and coming up, and don't lurch upward—let your quadriceps stand you up smoothly. This exercise is done on the balls of the feet; your heels will rise up off the floor, naturally.

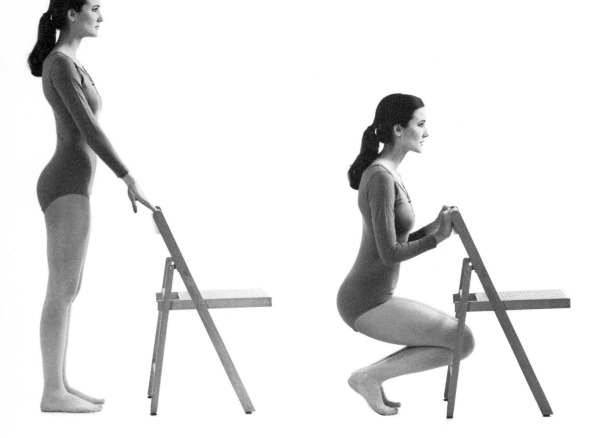

Legs and Buttocks

23. Alternating Step-ups:
One set.
Ten repetitions with each leg.

Another good exercise for sports, this one tones the buttocks as well as the quadriceps.

Stand in front of a stool or bench that is a foot and a half to two feet high. Put your right foot on it and step up for one repetition. Now step down with your right foot, leave your left foot on the bench, and step up on it for one repetition with the other leg. Do ten with each; and step up, don't lunge.

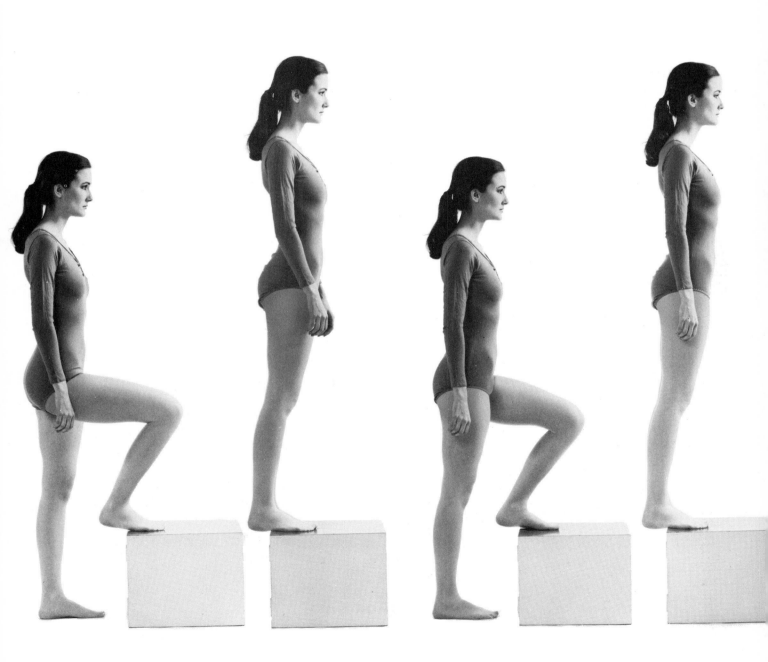

Legs and Buttocks

24. Lying Rear Leg Raises:
One set.
Ten repetitions with each leg.

A fine flexibility exercise and good for people with bad lower backs, this is primarily for hardening the buttocks and hips.

Lie on your stomach, your upper body raised and supported on your elbows. Raise your right leg up behind you as far as you can without bending much at the knee, then lower it to the floor. Do ten with the right leg, then ten with the left.

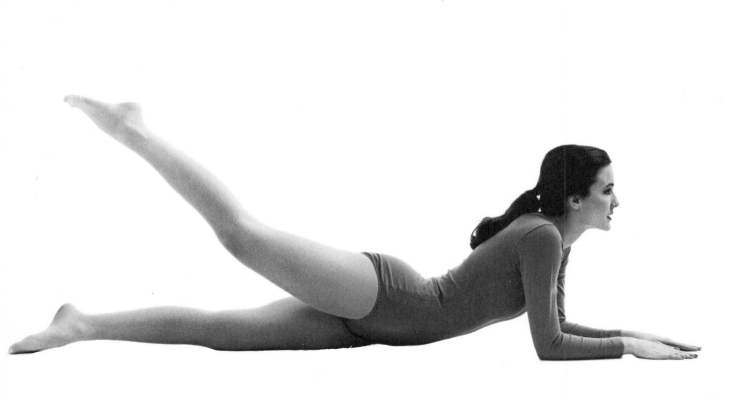

Legs and Buttocks

25. One-Leg Calf Raises:
One set.
Twenty repetitions with each leg.

In this calf-raise exercise, the movement is isolated in one calf at a time.

Find something like a few books or a rock, six inches thick or so, to stand on with the ball and instep of your right foot, letting your heel hang off the back, thereby extending the calf muscle. You might want to hold onto something in front of you for balance, but don't use it to pull yourself up. Now stand up on the toes of your right foot. Go as high as you can, feel the calf stretch, and hold it there for a count of two before coming down. Do twenty raises with your right leg, then twenty with your left.

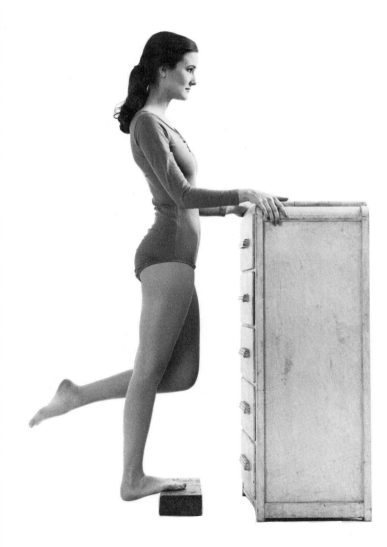
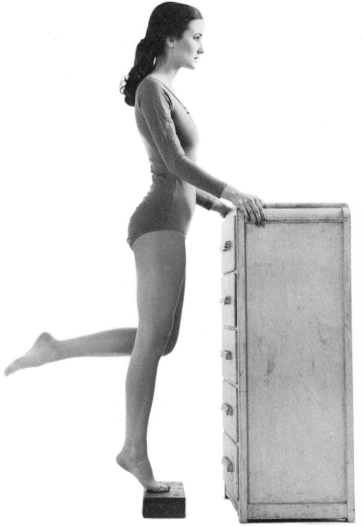

Chest

26. Push-ups:
One set.
Twenty repetitions.

Push-ups tone the pectoral muscles of the chest, and also the shoulders and the backs of the arms. To get much benefit from them you have to do them correctly. Here's how:

Start with your hands on a level with your chest and a little more than shoulder width apart. Lift your waist from the floor so that only your chest is touching. Now, keeping your head down and your back straight, push up until your arms are fully extended.

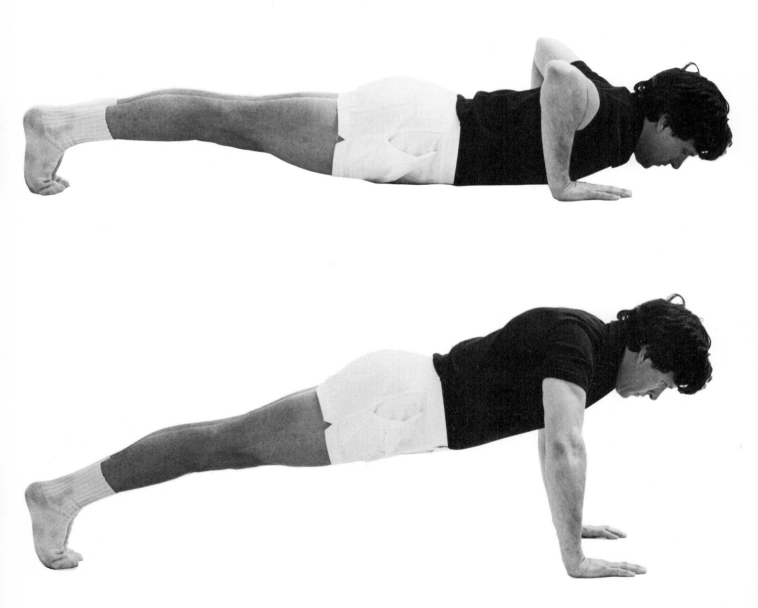

Chest

**26A. Alternate Exercise:
Bent-Knee Push-ups:**
One set.
Twenty repetitions.

Standard push-ups are often difficult for women. Here is an alternate way of doing them that is of almost equal toning benefit.

Start with your chin touching the floor, your weight resting on your hands and knees, your hands approximately shoulder width apart. Push up and back, keeping your back and waist in a straight line, to a crawling position, for one repetition.

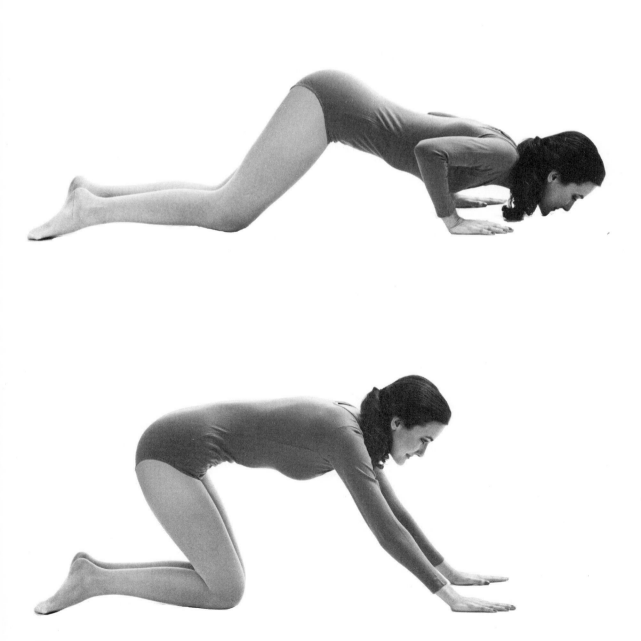

Chest

27. Prone Flies:
One set.
Twenty repetitions.

Flies not only tone but shape the pectoral muscles. They are excellent for swimmers, huggers, and anyone who wants a firm, high chest.

Lie on your back. Holding a large book or something of comparable weight in each hand, stretch your arms out perpendicular to your body and lift them an inch or two off the floor—they should not touch the ground at the end of each rep. Now bring your arms up toward each other, keeping them in a slight bow as if you were hugging a tree, until the books touch. Tense your chest at the top, then lower your arms slowly, keeping the strain on your pectorals.

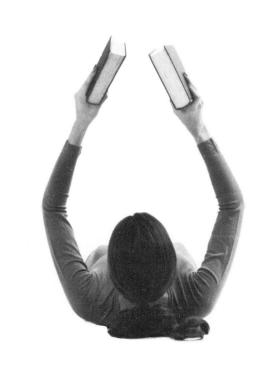

Back

28. Lower-Back Extensions:
One set.
Ten repetitions.

This extension is similar to but a bit harder than Exercise 11 in Program One. Like it, this is a fine flexibility exercise, good for tennis players, climbers, skiers, swimmers and runners, and can be helpful to lower-back problems, as it concentrates on the erector muscles around the base of the spine.

Lie on your stomach with your feet against something that won't move and your hands held together at the small of your back. Now, arching at the waist, bring your upper body up as far as you can; hold it at maximum extension for a count of two, then slowly lower it again for one repetition.

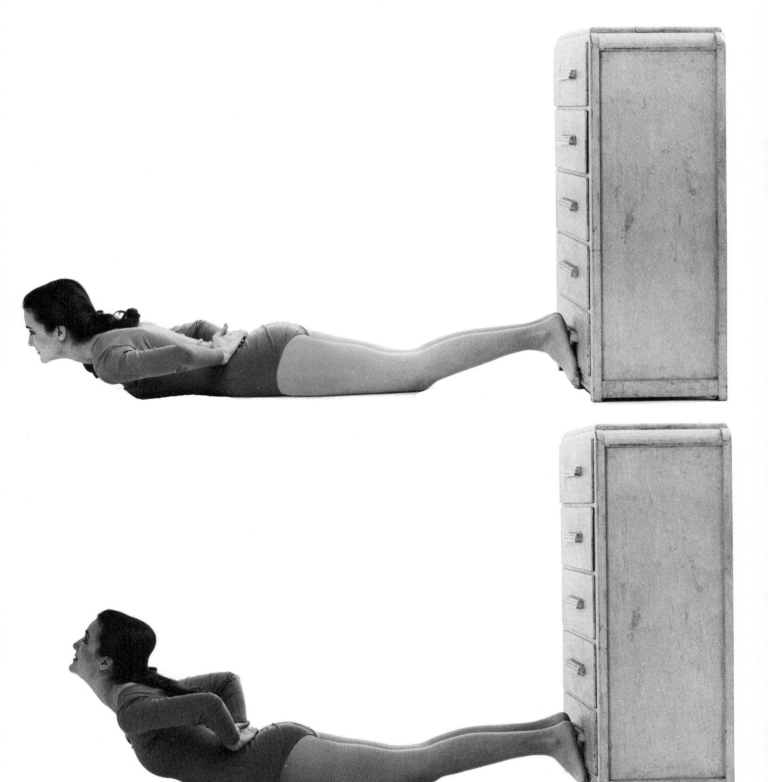

Back

29. Doorknob Pulls:
One set.
Twenty repetitions.

As far as I know I invented this exercise—on the bathroom door of a motel in northern Iowa. Whether I did or not, it's a beauty when done right and a back-wrenching dog when it's not. You can do it on almost anything that is immovable and about waist high, but I'll describe it for you using a door. A sturdy door.

Open the door halfway. Put your feet on either side of it at the bottom, heels together. Now take hold of both knobs and lean back, bowing at the waist. Without moving your legs, pull yourself straight across and touch the door with your chest. Your waist should remain bowed and your chest in the same plane as you approach and touch the door, then let yourself back out slowly. And your back, not your arms, should do the pulling: If you feel it much in your arms you are doing it wrong.

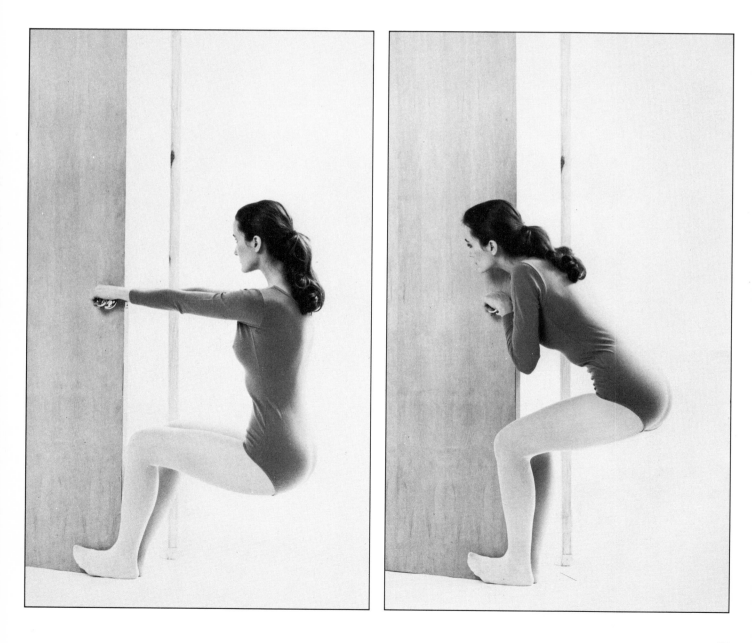

Shoulders

30. Push-offs:
One set.
Twenty repetitions.

Look back at the push-offs in Program One (Exercise 13). Do this exercise in exactly the same way, with your hands spaced a little wider than your shoulders, except here move your feet back farther from the object you are pushing off of, and put them together. This makes the exercise considerably harder, as well as locating it more in the rear deltoids, which generally need more toning than the front of the shoulders.

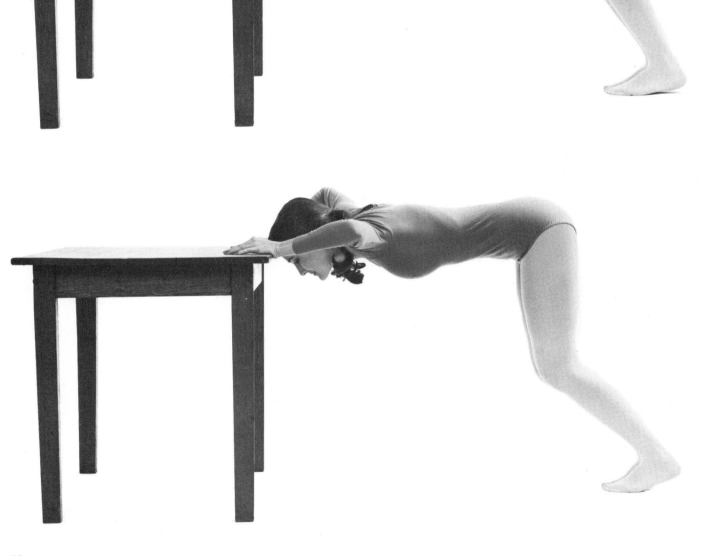

Shoulders

31. Standing Front and Lateral Flies:
One set.
Twenty repetitions with each arm.

This exercise shapes and hardens the shoulders and is good for all kinds of sports, notably cross-country skiing, in which poling is largely a function of the deltoid muscles being worked here.

Standing, hold two books (or other light objects) at your hips. Lift your right arm out to the side, to head level, keeping the arm straight; now lower it to your hip again and lift it up in front of you to head level. Lower it again for one repetition. Alternate right and left arms for twenty repetitions with each, and during each make your shoulder do the pulling; feel and isolate the strain there.

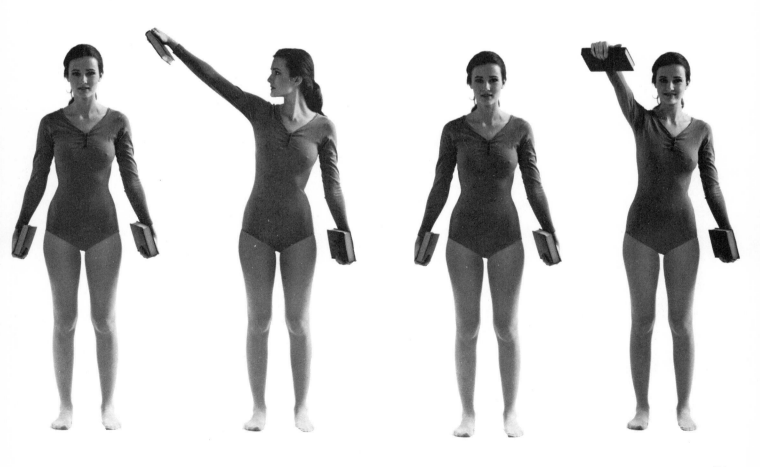

32. Isometric Doorknob Curls:
One set.
Ten repetitions.

Resistance here is achieved by holding muscle tension against an unmoving object. A door with a knob on either side is perfect for this exercise.

Standing close to the door, put a hand under either knob and take hold of it with the palm facing up. Keep your back straight. Pull upward on both knobs at the same time, as if you were trying to lift the door to the ceiling. Hold your maximum tension for three seconds and then relax, for one repetition.

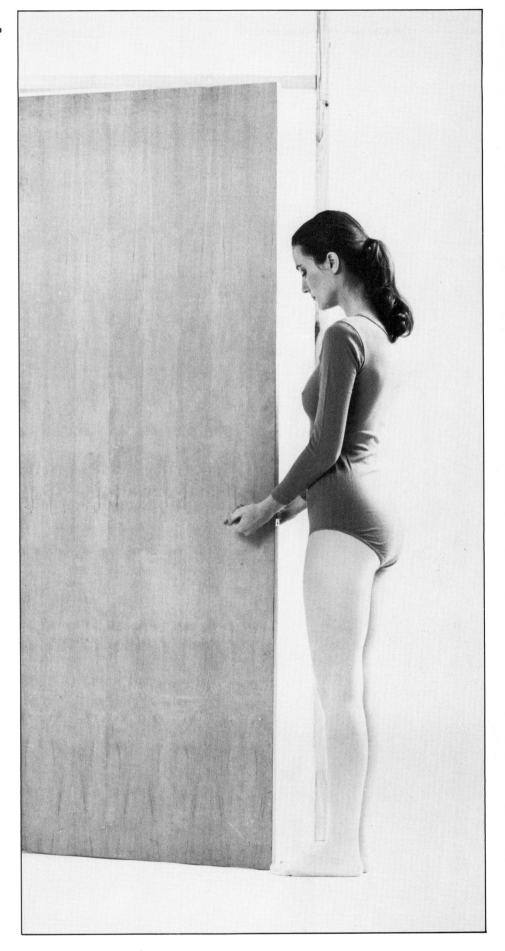

Arms

33. Triceps Push-offs:
One set.
Twenty repetitions.

This is a more difficult variation of the triceps exercise in Program One (*see* Exercise 16).

In this one the feet are together and farther away from the object. As in the beginner push-off, you should hold your back flat, and when your head touches the backs of your hands, your elbows should be pointed straight at the floor. You should feel all the resistance of the movement in the rear of your arms as opposed to your shoulders.

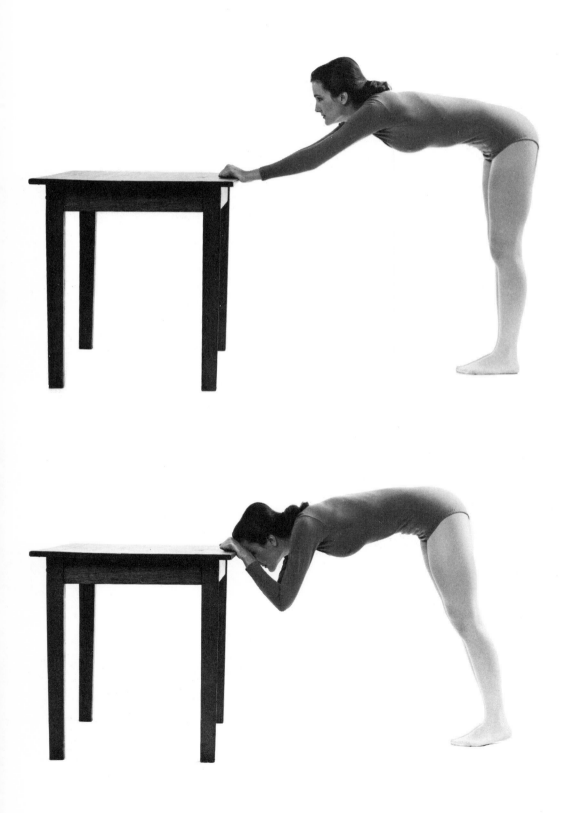

Program Three
(Advanced)
Target Time:
Twenty-nine minutes

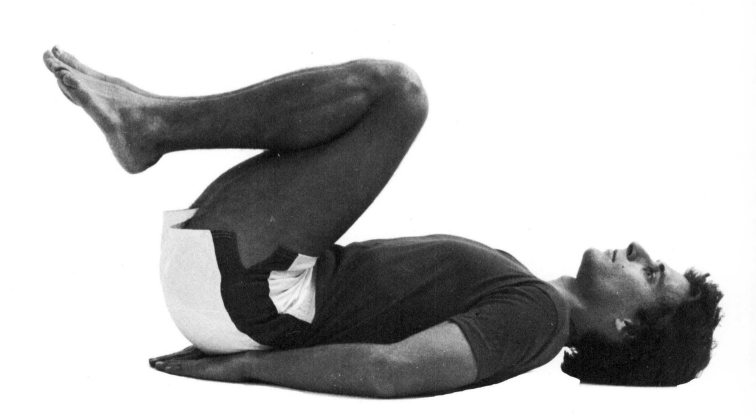

Waist

34. Bent-Leg Sit-ups:
One set.
One hundred repetitions.

One hundred of these three times a week will keep your upper abdomen toned and hard. The exercise is basically the same as the one shown in Exercise 17 of Program Two, except that in order to put more direct stress on the abdominals you should clasp your hands on your chest for this one. Touch your lower back to the floor on each repetition, and do the set fast.

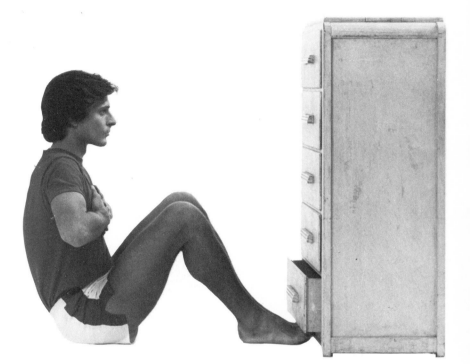

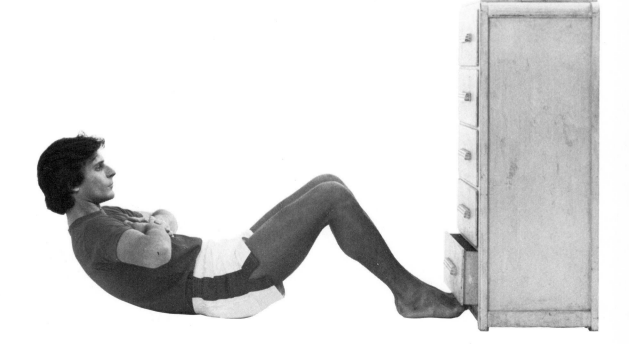

Waist

35. Leg-ins:
One set.
Fifty repetitions.

This is one of the best exercises there is for keeping a roll of soft off your lower abdomen. Like other lower-abdominal exercises it is also good for lower-back problems.

Lie on your back with your hands under your hips. Lift your legs six inches off the floor. Bring your knees in to your chest, then stretch your legs out straight again for one repetition. Don't let your feet or legs touch the floor throughout the set.

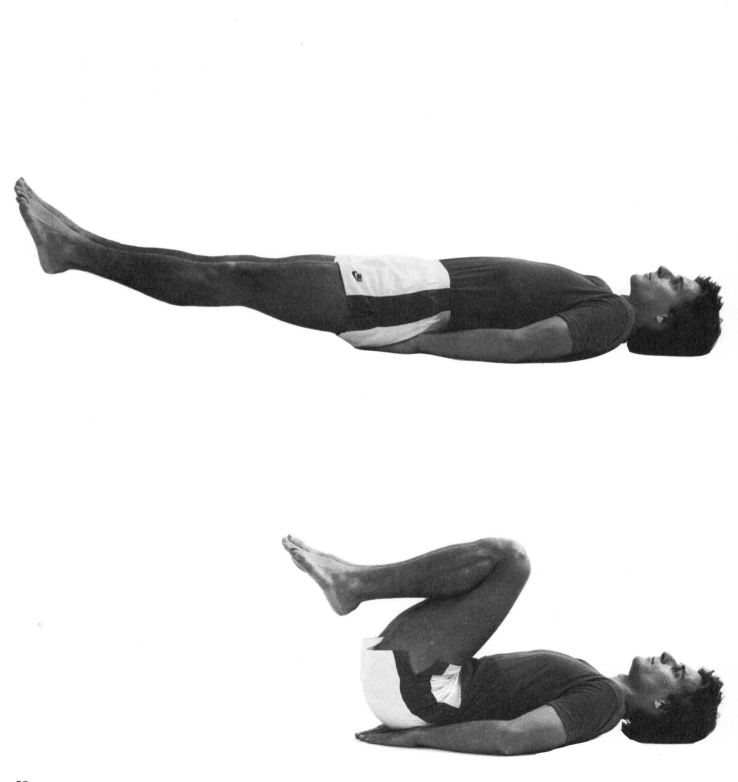

Waist

36. Crunches:
One set.
Twenty-five repetitions.

When done correctly, this is an excellent all-around waist-toning exercise and is also good for increasing flexibility in the upper spine.

Lie on your back with your legs bent steeply at the knees and elevated, and your hands on your hips. Lifting your shoulders from the floor, touch your chin to your chest and "crunch" or tense your stomach muscles as you do it.

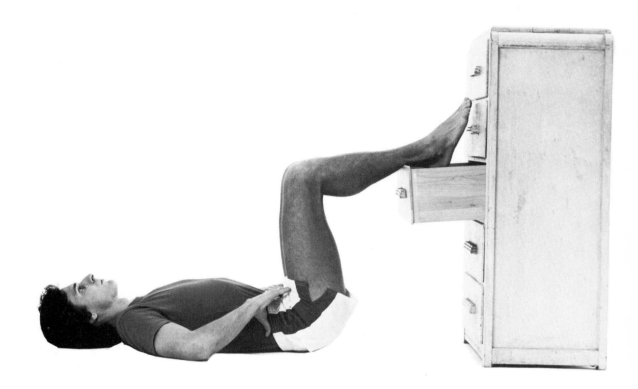

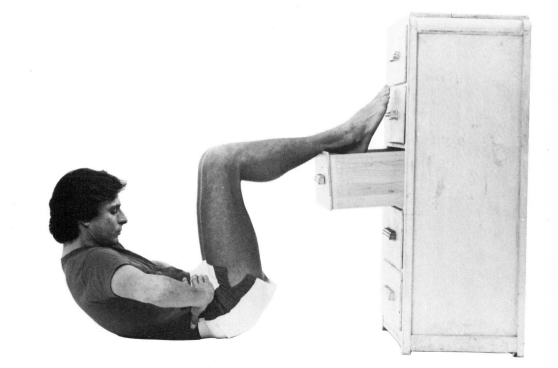

Waist

37. Side Bends:
One set.
Thirty repetitions to each side.

This exercise is practically the same as the one in Program Two shown in Exercise 19. In this one hold a book, or object of similar weight, in the dropping arm, and do thirty reps to each side instead of twenty. Do them as fast as you can without bouncing.

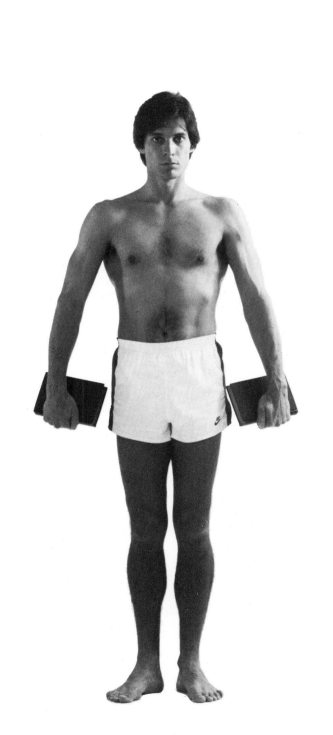
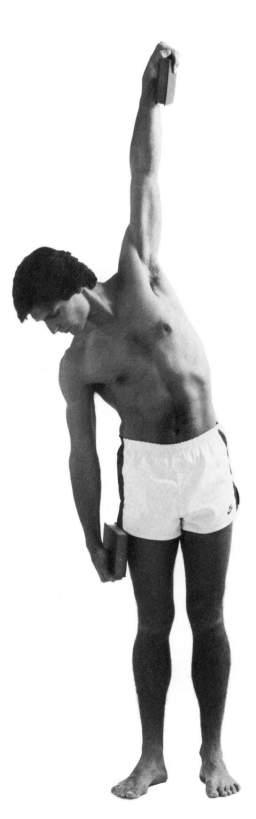

Waist

38. Seated Twists:
One set.
Fifty repetitions to each side.

Good for spinal flexibility, and very good for hardening the intercostal and oblique muscles of the waist.

Sit in a chair holding two books with your arms out to your sides. You should face forward throughout the exercise. Twist at the waist to your right, bringing your arms and upper body around as far as they will go. Then come back to your starting position and twist in the other direction. Alternate fifty repetitions to each side, and do them fast.

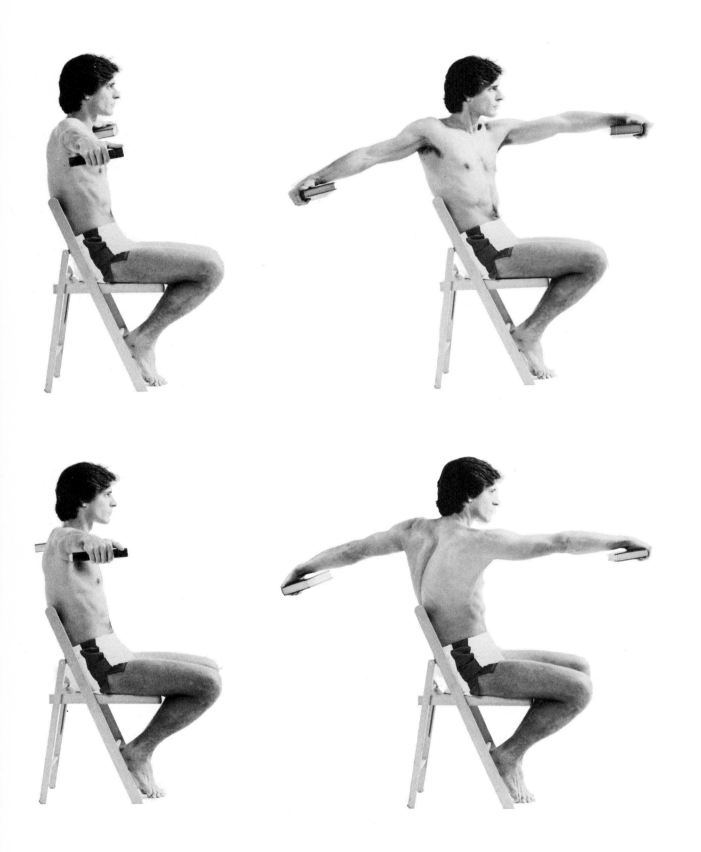

Waist

39. Back Bends:
One set.
Ten repetitions.

If you get a stiff lower back from time to time, this is a good way to help it. It is also good for tightening and hardening all the major muscles of the waist.

In this exercise each repetition is made up of three separate movements, all starting from the same position.

Stand with your feet shoulder width apart, your hands on your hips. Bend straight backward at the waist as far as you comfortably can, then pull upright, using your stomach muscles. Now bend backward at an angle to the right and pull upright. Finally, for one full repetition, bend backward at an angle to the left and pull back up. Don't bounce up—make your abdominal muscles pull you.

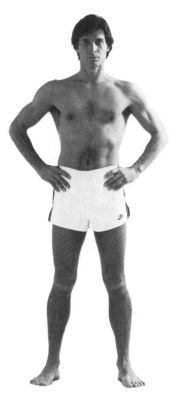
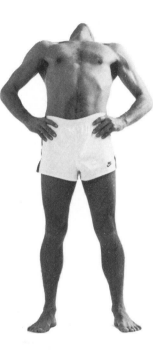
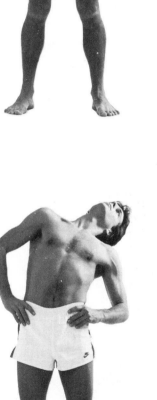
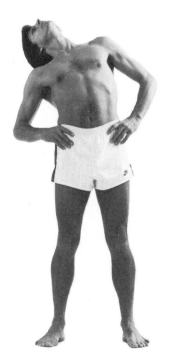
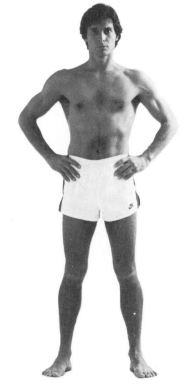

63

Legs and Buttocks

40. Knee Bends:
One set.
Thirty repetitions.

I worked out for myself this particular deep knee bend. It puts more stress on the quadriceps muscles than any one I know of. It has to be done strictly, and it might take you a few sets before you are doing it right. Done correctly, you will feel this exercise all through the front of your thighs.

Stand holding the two knobs of a door or something else that is lower than your waist. Turn your feet out, with your heels together, about twelve inches from the bottom of the door. When you go down, let your upper body swing out and back, away from the door, keeping your arms straight and letting your knees move in toward the door. Now stand up from that position—making the fronts of your thighs do all the work—for one repetition.

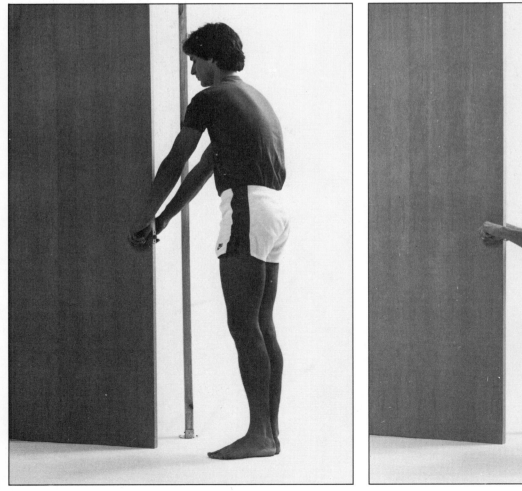

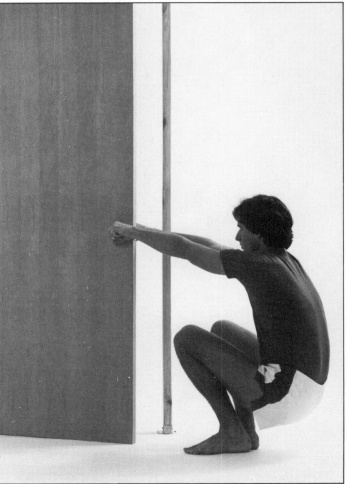

Legs and Buttocks

41. Lunges:

One set.
Fifteen repetitions with each leg.

Lunges tone the upper legs and hips. Because they strengthen the quadriceps and improve balance and flexibility as well, they are an excellent exercise for sports.

Stand with your feet together and your arms held out at your side for balance. Now step forward two to three feet with your right leg and sink on it until you touch the knee of your left leg to the floor. Come back up to your original position for one rep with the right leg. Alternate legs for fifteen repetitions with each.

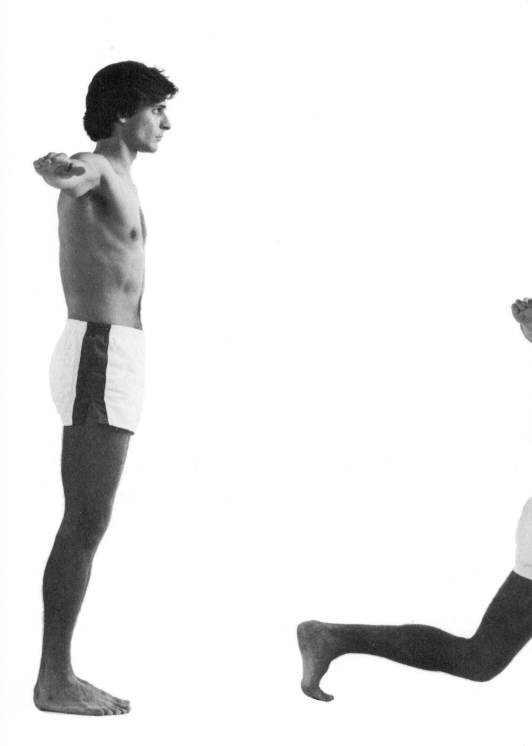

Legs and Buttocks

42. Leg Curls:
One set.
Fifteen repetitions with each leg.

Leg curls work on the biceps femoris muscles at the backs of the thighs. This particular leg curl is one I developed; it depends for its effectiveness entirely on concentration.

From a standing position, bend over and hold onto something lower than your hips. Slowly, imagining it weighted, curl your left leg by bringing your heel up toward your buttocks. Your knee should be pointed directly at the floor throughout the repetition. This is a self-resistant exercise: you must produce, by concentration, a counterforce to the movement of the exercise; you do that by flexing the muscle at the back of your leg and imagining that you are drawing the leg up against a weight or force that barely allows it to move. The burn in your hamstring will let you know if you are doing it correctly.

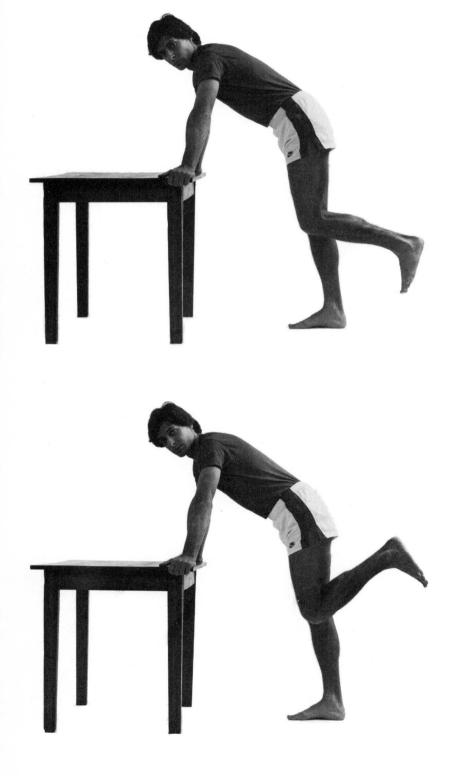

Legs and Buttocks

43. Calf Raises:
One set.
Repetitions as specified below.

This is a whole routine of calf raises in one set; it and a little walking every once in a while is all the toning your calves will ever need.

Take the same position, with your feet on a book or ledge, as shown in Exercise 8. Do twenty of the two-leg calf raises described there, holding each at the top for two seconds. Now, without resting, do twenty with just the right leg, then twenty with the left. To finish off, stand on your tiptoes and alternately relax and flex your calves twenty times—each flex should be held until the calves ache.

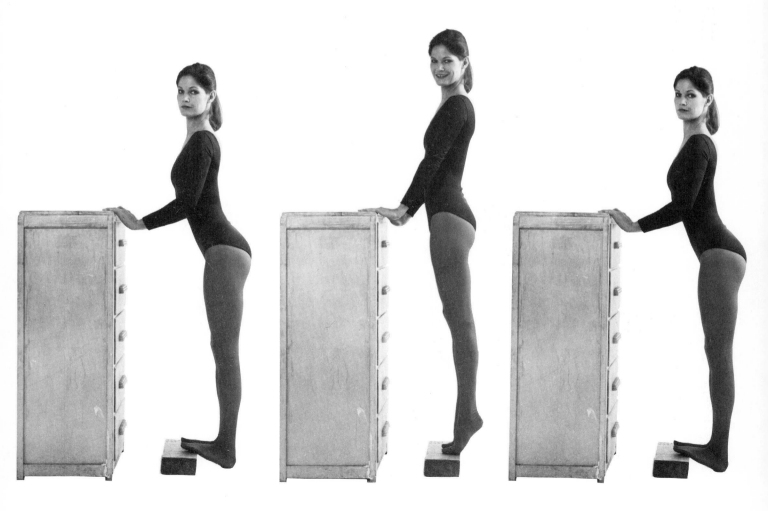

Chest

44. Push-ups:
One set.
Twenty-five repetitions.

This is a more difficult variation of the ordinary push-up. Because your body is going lower than your hands, more of the pectoral muscle is being reached and toned.

Put your feet up on something that is approximately the same height as the two chairs (or benches, or blocks, etc.) you are pushing up from. Let your body down so that your chest drops below your hands, and push back up until your arms are fully extended. Hold your back straight through the repetition.

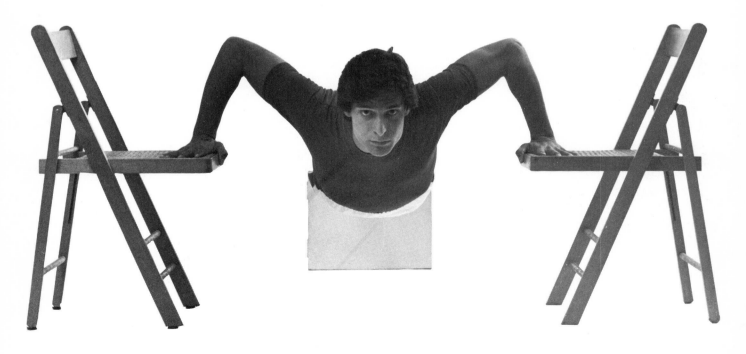

Chest

45. Alternate Flies and Pull-overs:
One set.
Twenty-five repetitions.

This one exercise when done in good form will harden the pectoral and serratus muscles of the chest and also help to tone the intercostals and upper abdominals. It is very good for upper-body flexibility.

Lie on a bench—or something else less wide than your shoulders and long enough to accommodate your back and hips—holding two heavy books, or objects of similar weight, directly over your chest. With your arms slightly bent, lower the books out to the sides until they pass beneath the plane of your chest; then bring your arms back up in a slight bow, as though you were hugging something, until the books touch; then, with the books together, lower your arms back behind your head as far as they will go; and finally, using your chest and upper-stomach muscles, pull them back to vertical for one repetition of the exercise. Try to do the four movements smoothly and with maximum stretch.

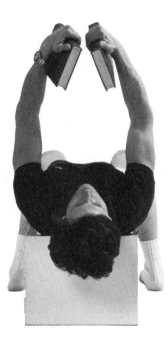

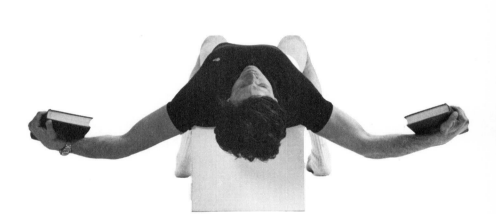

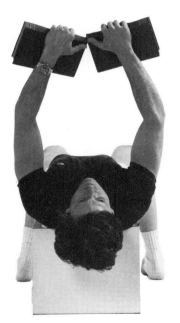

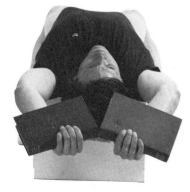

Back

46. Pull-ups:
One set.
Twenty-five repetitions.

These pull-ups tone most of the muscles of the upper back, particularly the latissimus dorsi. To do them you will need a couple of stable objects about two feet high—chairs are fine—and a broomstick, or some other kind of sturdy pole.

Lie on your back between the two chairs (which should be four to five feet apart) and take a wide grip on the pole stretched between them. Keeping your heels on the floor, pull your chest as close as you can to the pole (ideally, it should touch it), then let yourself down slowly for one repetition. Keep your body straight as you do these, and make your back do the pulling.

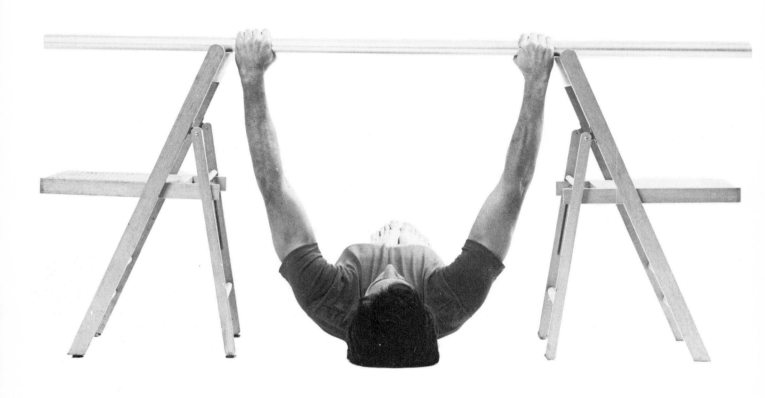

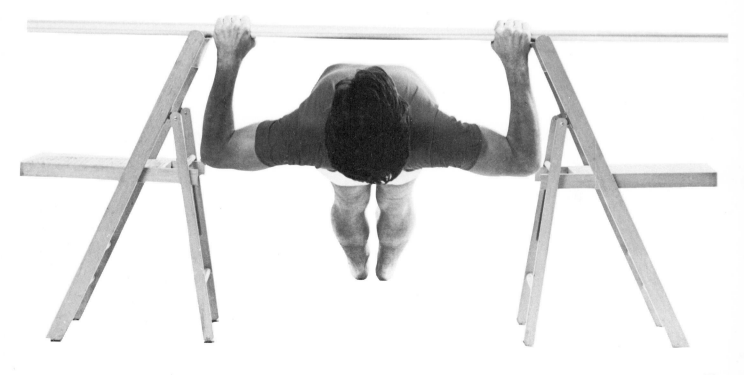

Back

47. Lower-Back Extensions:
One set.
Twenty repetitions.

Primarily for the spinal erector muscles, this exercise also tones the buttocks. It is a great exercise for your tennis or squash game, and for cross-country skiing.

Lie on your stomach and chest with your head off the floor, your arms lifted behind you and to the sides. Curl your legs and upper body up toward each other—leaving only your stomach and hips on the floor—as far as they will go, and hold them there for three seconds before relaxing, for one repetition.

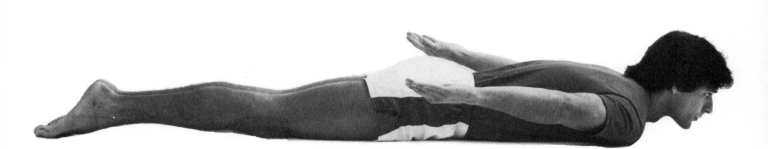

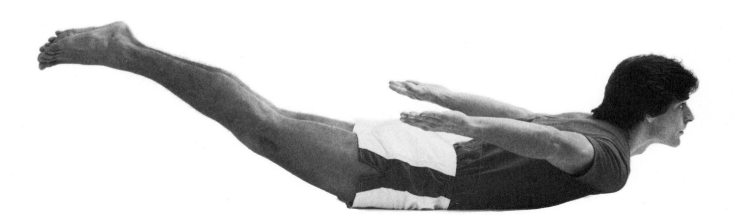

Shoulders

48. Isometric Doorway Presses:
One set.
Twenty repetitions.

Presses are for toning the deltoid muscles of the shoulders. The press shown here is isometric, or static.

Stand in a doorway; if you can't reach the top of the doorway with your arms still bent, stand on a chair. Hold your feet shoulder width apart; put your palms on the top of the doorway and push upward, facing forward. Hold each press at maximum tension for three seconds.

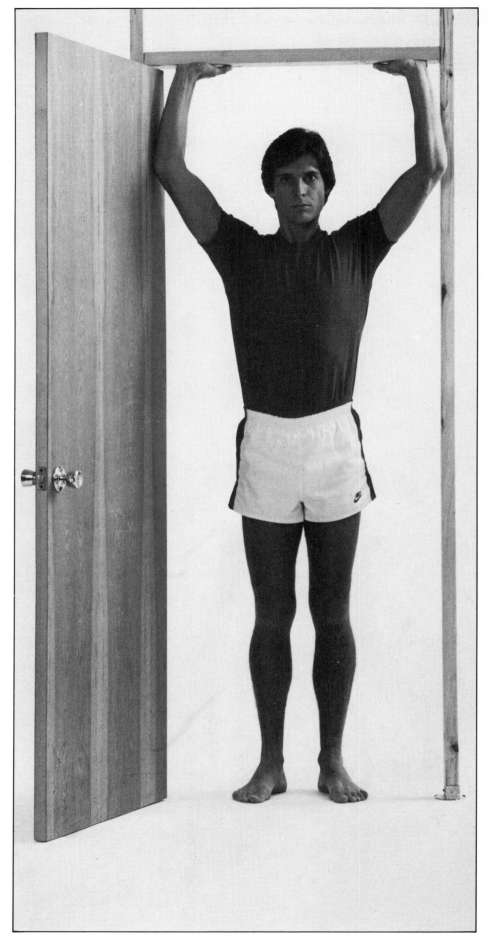

Shoulders

48A. Alternate Exercise: Headstand Presses:
One set.
Ten repetitions.

This is an excellent free-form exercise for both toning and flexibility—but your shoulders will have to be in very good shape to do it even once.

Go into a headstand close enough to a wall so that your heels touch it. Your hands should be on the floor in line with your head and spaced a bit wider than your shoulders. Arch your back and push straight up until your arms are fully extended for one repetition.

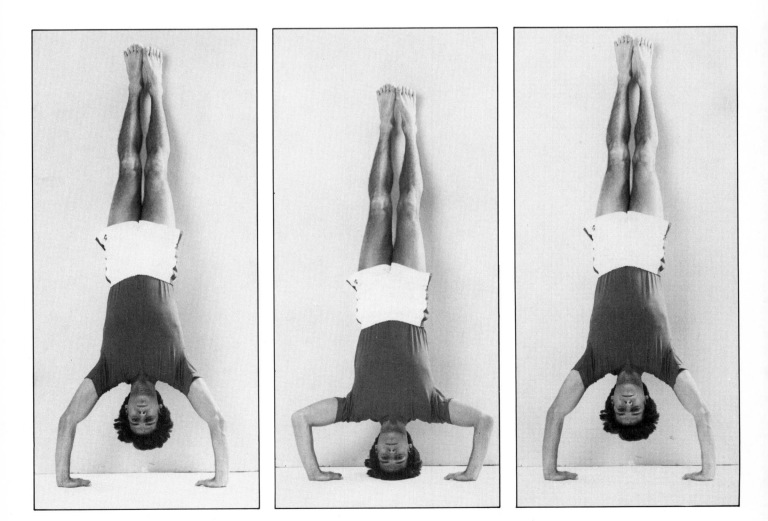

Shoulders

49. Isometric Doorway Flies:
One set.
Twenty repetitions.

In this exercise for the deltoids and trapezius muscles of the shoulders you will again be using a doorway to push against. As in the previous exercise, the toning effect is achieved by the resistance of the doorway to the muscular force you exert against it.

With your feet shoulder width apart, press the backs of your hands against the doorway and push outward and up. Hold each repetition at maximum tension for three seconds.

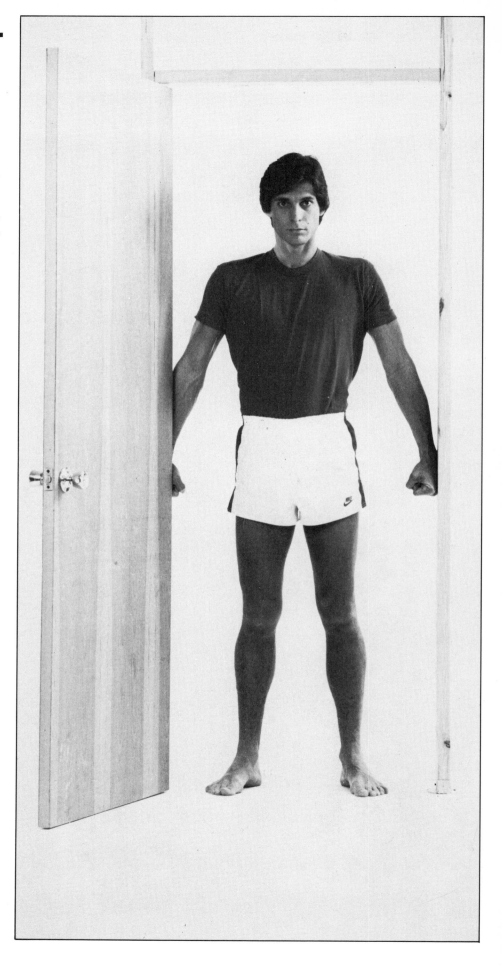

Arms

50. Curls:
One set.
Twenty repetitions with each arm.

The resistance is against yourself in this exercise for the biceps, and concentration is particularly important.

Sit or kneel with your left leg extended and cross your right arm over it at the elbow. The arm should be extended, your hand near the floor. Now take hold of your right arm near the wrist with your left hand. As you curl your right fist up toward your chin, put enough pressure on your right arm with your left hand so that it really has to work to rise.

Do twenty reps with the right arm, then reverse your position and do twenty with the left.

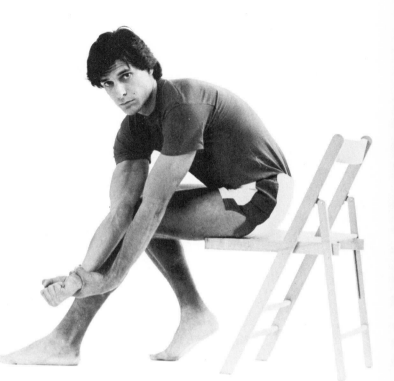

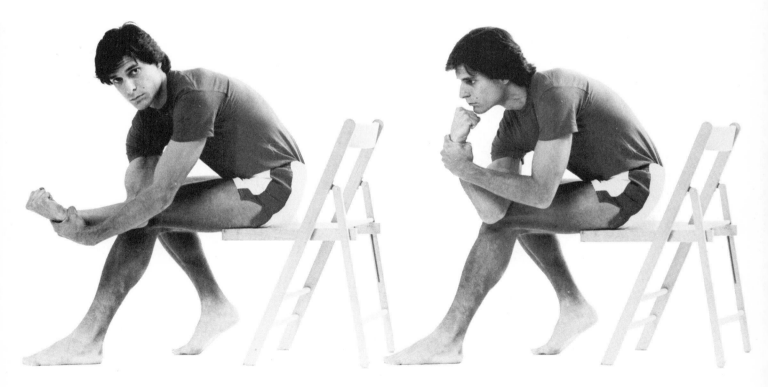

Arms

51. Dips:
One set.
Twenty repetitions.

This particular dip is designed to tone the triceps muscles at the backs of your arms. If you find you are unable to do twenty repetitions, do the alternate exercise instead.

Put your feet together on something about chair height and support your upper body, arms extended and knuckles facing forward, on something slightly higher. Now let your seat sink toward the floor until your chest is on a plane with your hands, and push smoothly back up. Keep your legs straight and don't let them help push you up.

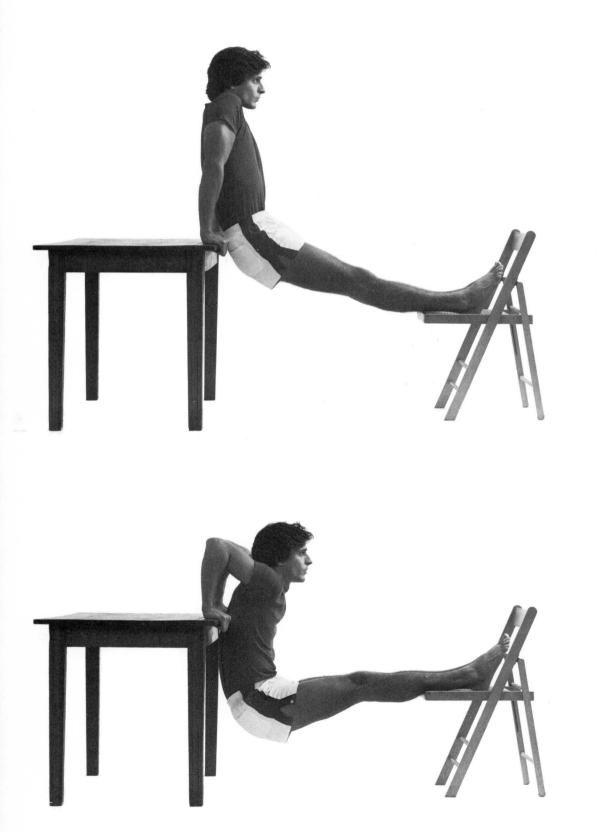

This alternate dip is easier because your feet are on the floor, rather than elevated, and closer to your body. The dip is done in the same way as the one above, and, again, you shouldn't push with your legs, but let the backs of your arms do the work.

51A. Alternate Exercise: Dips with Feet on Floor:
One set.
Twenty repetitions.

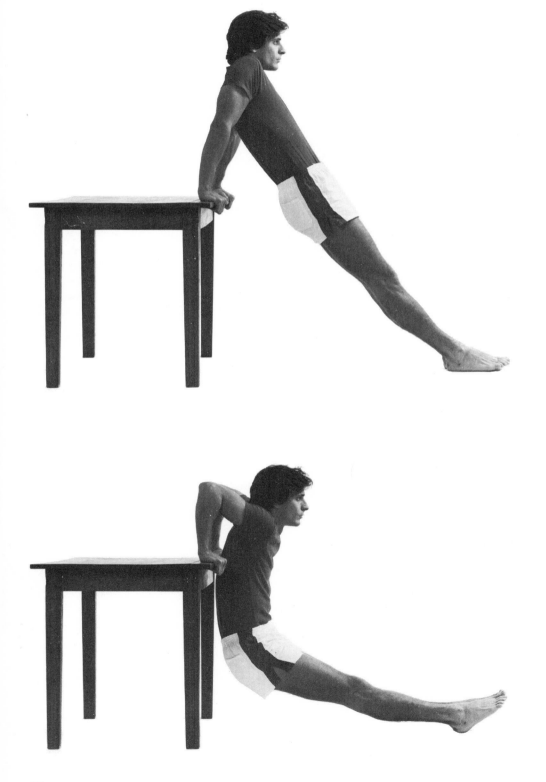

Section II: Exercises with Weights

This second section was developed for people who like training with weights. The equipment requirements are simple and cheap: all you need for these exercises are two dumbbells, a barbell, and a bench. The exercises can be done in a gym, though they were designed to be done right at home. You could even travel with them, I suppose, if you really wanted to. I used to know a guy who hitchhiked all over the country carrying 150 pounds of weights in a laundry bag.

The programs here will not give you big muscles. If you want big muscles there are plenty of books available that will tell you how to get them with weights, including ones by my friends Arnold Schwarzenegger, Frank Zane, and Franco Columbo. The weight programs here are for toning and hardening the muscles, not for building them. For toning you want a lot of repetitions and only enough weight to reach, work, and "burn" the muscles, and that is not very much weight—no matter how big and strong you are. I am fairly big and strong myself, and when I do these exercises I use two twenty-pound dumbbells and a forty-pound barbell. If my wife Patricia, who is five feet four and weighs 120 pounds, were to do them (she doesn't), she would probably use five-pound dumbbells and a fifteen-pound barbell.

To determine how much weight you should use, do this:

Put twenty-five pounds on a bar and do twenty quick bench presses, as described in Program Five (Exercise 74). If you can't do twenty, take off weight until you can—comfortably, but with the slight burning sensation in your chest that lets you know you have reached and worked the muscles there. If twenty-five pounds feels ridiculously light, add weight until, after twenty reps, you get the right sensation. You are *not* trying to find the maximum amount of weight you can do twenty-five repetitions with—that amount would build your chest—but your proper toning poundage, which is considerably less. I would do the twenty bench presses here, for example, with forty pounds: I *could* do them with two hundred. To determine how much weight you should use on the dumbbells, start with fifteen pounds on each and experiment with the curls shown in Program Five (Exercise 80) in the same way.

Once you can do the advanced program here within its Target Time, you might want to increase your weight for some if not all of the exercises, but it isn't necessary. Here, as in the other two sections, it is the design of the exercises, high repetitions, good form, and concentration that keep you hard, not more and more weight.

Remember to do the exercises in good form, as they are described, and to breathe properly.

Program Four
(Beginner)
Target Time:
Twenty-one Minutes

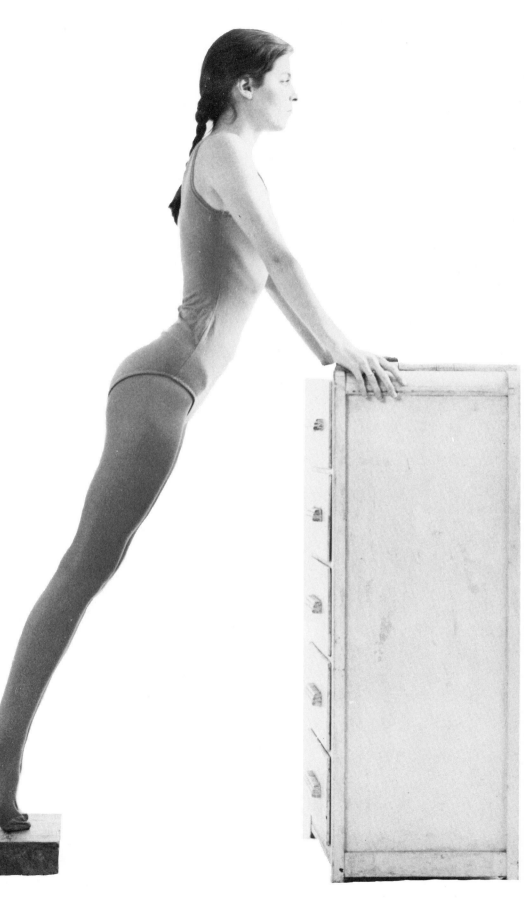

Waist

52. Sit-ups:
One set.
Fifteen repetitions

I got this sit-up from my buddy Jim Lynch, who uses it in his aerobics class. Anyone can do it, and it's an excellent upper-abdominal hardener.

Lie on your back, arms extended behind your head, legs bent. Raise your upper body, with your arms over your head, and close the sit-up by dropping your head between your knees and clapping the floor with your hands. Try not to throw yourself up, but let the muscles of your stomach raise you.

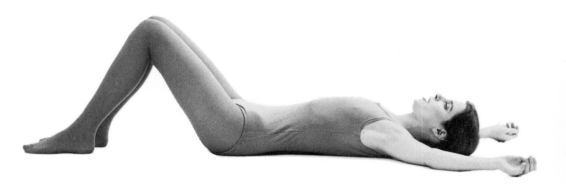

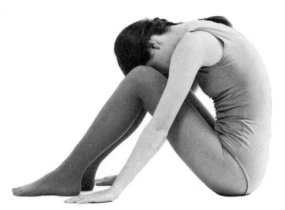

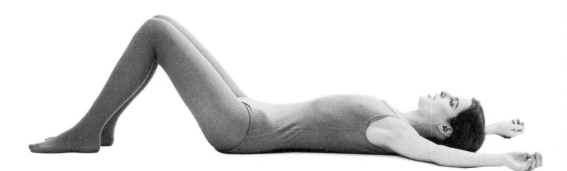

Waist

53. Alternating Knee-ins:
One set.
Fifteen repetitions with each leg.

This exercise concentrates on the lower abdominals. It too is good for lower-back problems and spinal flexibility. Bring your right knee as far in toward your chest as you can get it, extend it slowly back out again, and drop it to the floor for one repetition. Alternate legs for fifteen repetitions with each.

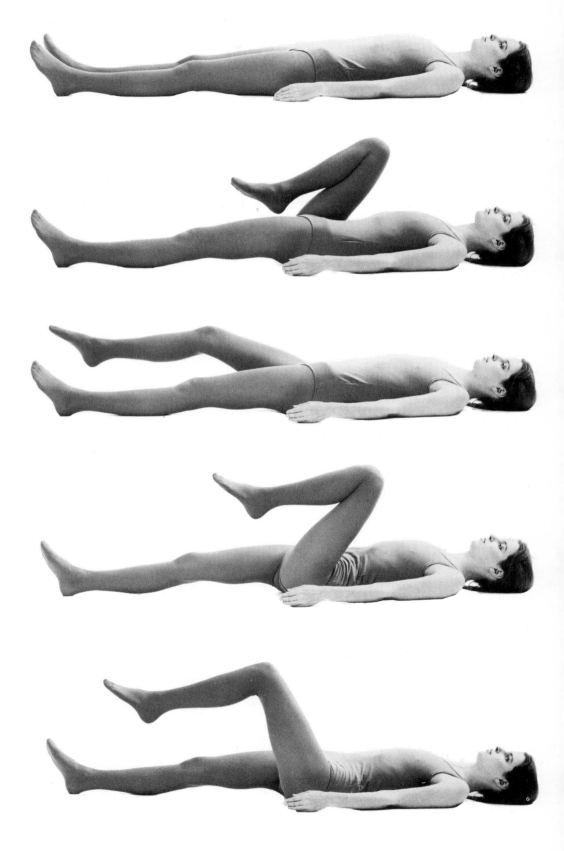

Waist

54. Torso Sweeps:
One set.
Fifteen repetitions.

This is a fine flexibility exercise as well as an excellent toner of the abdominal, oblique, and intercostal muscles. All tennis players, I believe, should warm up with sweeps, and people with bad lower backs should do them every morning.

Stand with your feet shoulder width apart and your hands clasped over your head. Bend at the waist to your right side, then sweep down and around, until you are bending straight ahead, then sweep up your left side. Make your stomach muscles really stretch out on both sides of the sweep.

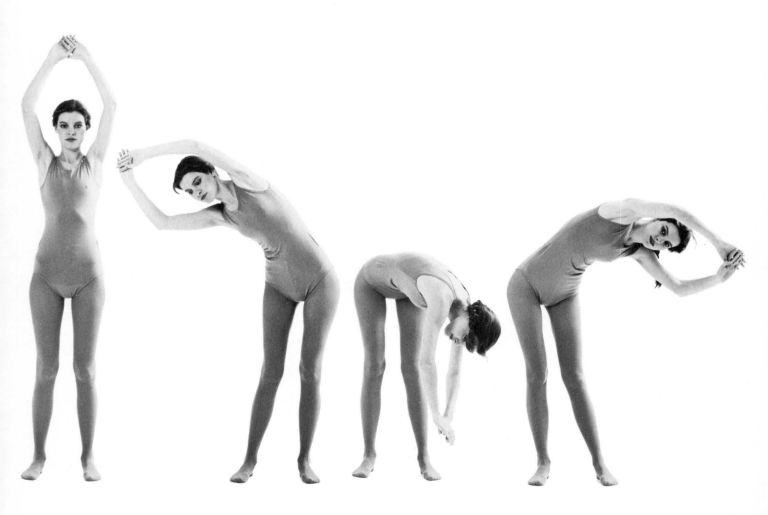

Legs and Buttocks

55. Standing Leg-outs:
One set.
Fifteen repetitions with each leg.

Leg-outs tone the hips and buttocks. For best results do them quickly and carry each repetition to a full extension.

Stand holding something at about hip height. Without turning your hips, raise your right leg out to the side as high as it will go, then lower it again. Do fifteen with that leg, then fifteen with the other.

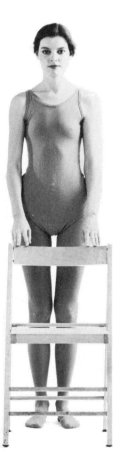

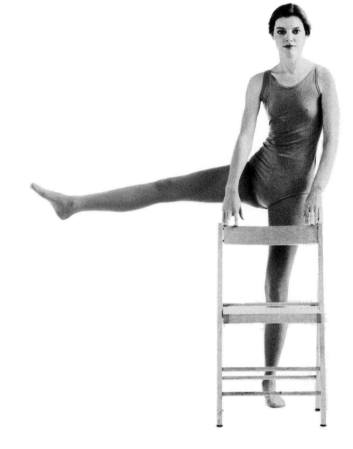

Legs and Buttocks

56. Step-ups:
One set.
Fifteen repetitions with each leg.

Step-ups harden the quadriceps muscles at the front of the upper thigh. They are a good exercise for almost all sports, particularly cross-country and downhill skiing.

Find a stool or a bench one to two feet high. Stand in front of it, holding a dumbbell in your left hand. Step up on the stool with your right foot (*step,* don't heave up—let the leg muscle bring you up). When you step down, onto your left foot, leave the right foot on the stool for fourteen more reps with that leg. Then put the dumbbell in your right hand and step up fifteen times on your left leg.

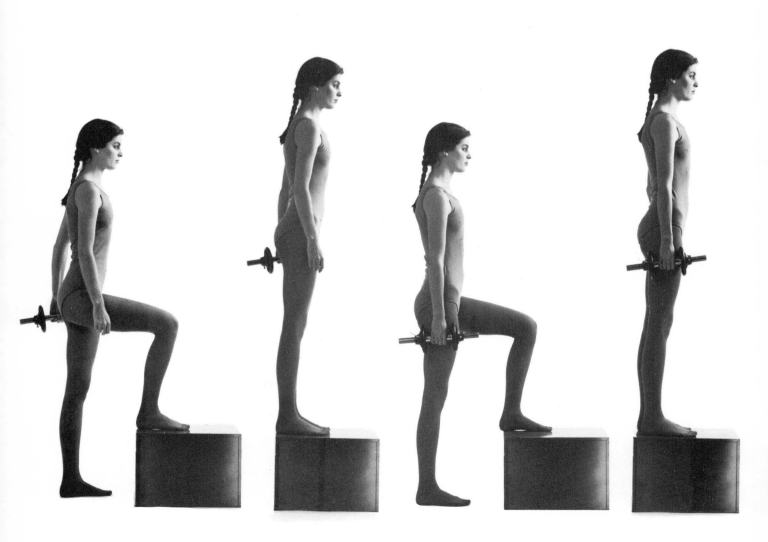

Legs and Buttocks

57. Bent-Over Calf Raises:
One set.
Fifteen repetitions.

For shaping and toning the calves. You *have* to do this one correctly to get any benefit from it.

Stand bent at the waist, your upper body leaning against something, your feet a few inches apart and a couple of feet behind your head. Your toes and the fronts of your insteps should be resting on a block or ledge, with your heels hanging off and down. Lower your heels until you feel the calves stretch; now stand up as far as you can on your toes, your upper body rocking forward as you do. Go up until your calves ache and hold the repetition there for a second or two before coming down.

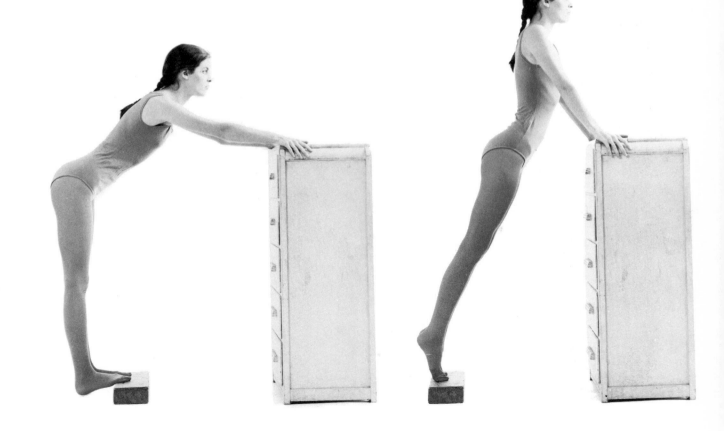

Chest

58. Prone Dumbbell Presses:
One set.
Fifteen repetitions with each arm.

This hardens and tones the pectoral muscles of the chest and is a particularly good exercise for women who are going slack there.

Lie on a bench holding the dumbbells at chest level with the near end of each bar touching your soulders. Press the dumbbell in your right hand and don't quite fully extend your arm, keeping tension on the chest muscle; now lower it slowly—don't drop it—and do a repetition with your left arm. Alternate for fifteen with each.

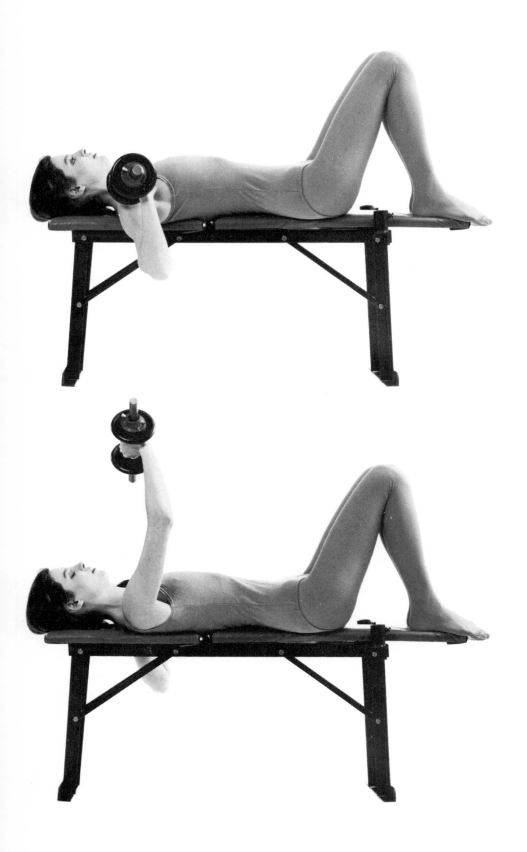

Chest

59. Dumbbell Pull-overs:
One set.
Fifteen repetitions.

This is good for your back and good for flexibility, and it tones your upper stomach as well as the serratus and lower pectoral muscles at which it is primarily directed.

Lie on the bench. Hold a dumbbell with both hands over your chest and a slight bend in your elbows. Keeping your arms bent slightly, lower the dumbbell behind your head as far as you are able, then bring it smoothly back up. Don't jerk it; raise it.

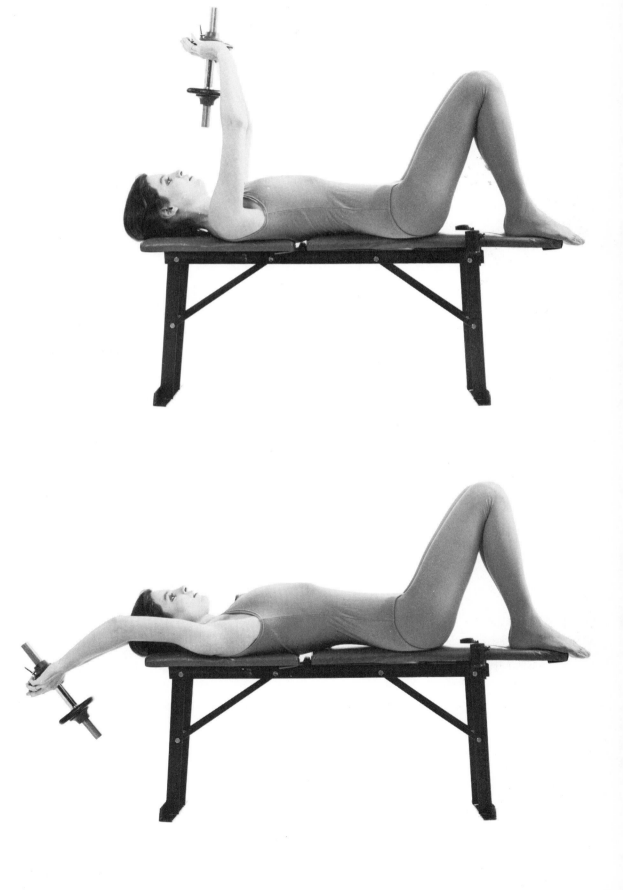

Back

60. Dumbbell Rows:
One set.
Fifteen repetitions with each arm.

This exercise has to be done strictly in order for it to reach the latissimus dorsi muscle of the back instead of the arms.

Stand bent over at the waist, your feet spread wide, your left hand on a bench or chair and your right holding a dumbbell off the ground. Now, feeling the exercise along the right side of your back—concentrating it there—lift the dumbbell up to touch your chest, then lower it smoothly. Do fifteen repetitions with that arm, then reverse your position and do fifteen with the left.

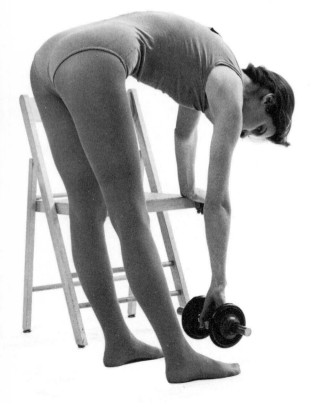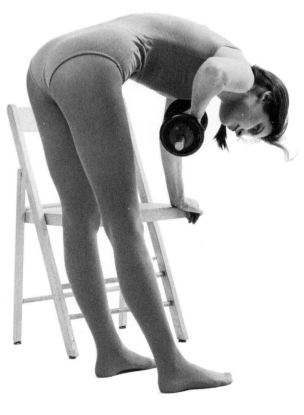

Back

61. Kick-backs:
One set.
Fifteen repetitions with each leg.

This exercise is very good for back problems and spinal flexibility. It not only tones the spinal erector muscles of the lower back, but hardens the buttocks as well.

Lie on your stomach on the bench. Arch your back by lifting your chest and head. Now kick your right leg up, bent slightly at the knee, as high as it will go, then lower it for one repetition. Do fifteen with the right leg, then fifteen with the left.

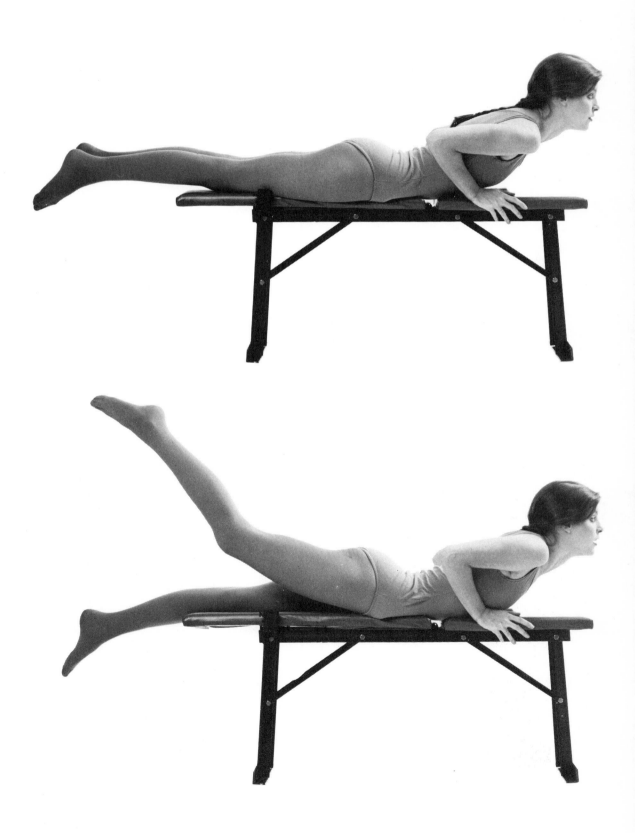

Shoulders

62. Standing Dumbbell Presses:
One set.
Fifteen repetitions with each arm.

This is for the deltoid muscles of the shoulders.

Stand with your feet twelve to eighteen inches apart, holding the two dumbbells at shoulder level. Keeping your back straight, press the dumbbell in your right hand to full extension of the arm, then lower it slowly. Alternate arms for fifteen reps apiece.

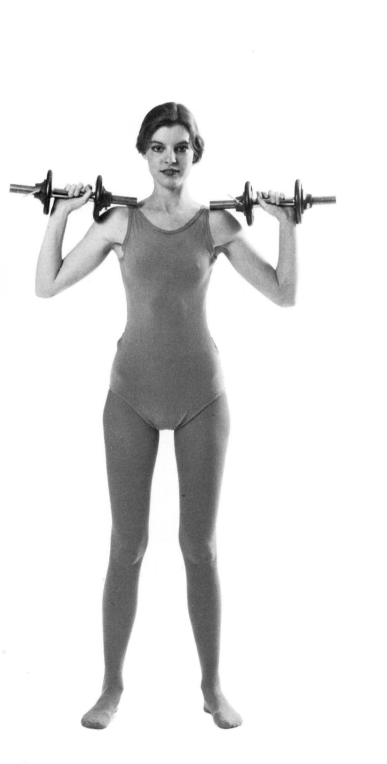

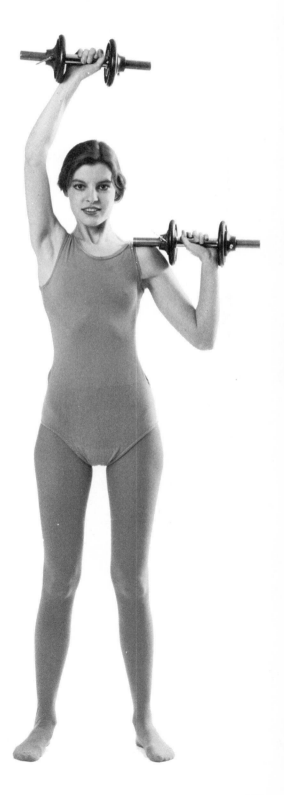

Shoulders

63. Front Dumbbell Raises:
One set.
Fifteen repetitions.

This exercise tones the trapezius muscles at the bottom of either side of the neck, and the frontal head, or section, of the deltoids.

Stand again with your feet approximately a foot and a half apart, holding a dumbbell between your legs. Keep your back straight and motionless as you raise the dumbbell directly overhead and then lower it again in one smooth motion.

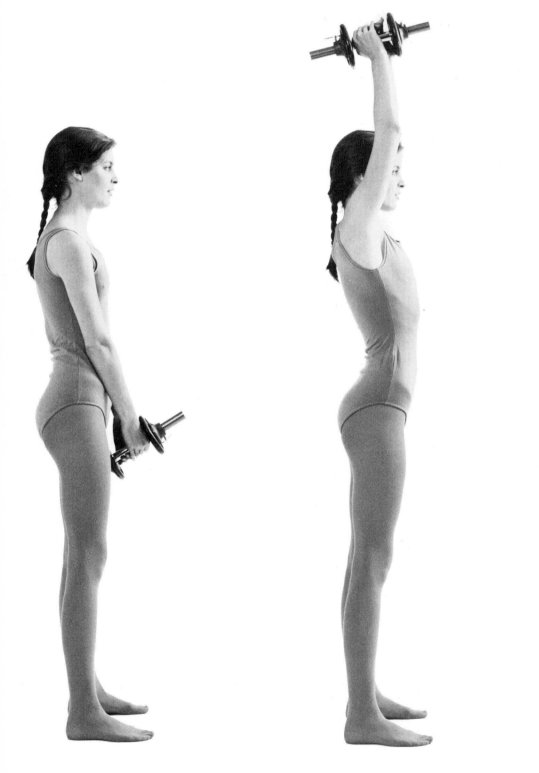
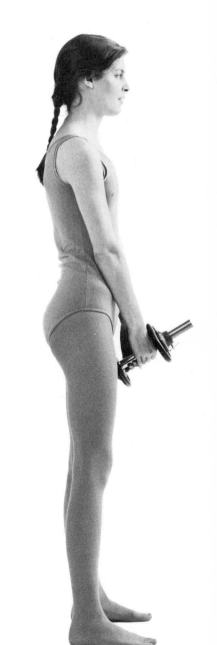

Arms

64. Standing Barbell Curls:
One set.
Fifteen repetitions.

This tones the biceps, the muscles at the front of your upper arms. It's a wonderful exercise for blue-fin tuna fishing, among other sports.

Stand with your feet comfortably apart, holding the barbell in front of you. Bend your elbows and bring the bar out from your hips an inch or two, just far enough to put tension on the biceps; this position will be the bottom of each repetition. Now without moving anything but your lower arms, curl the bar up toward your chest, but stop it before you lose tension on the biceps. Lower it slowly, for one repetition. When you start the curl, don't jerk the bar, bend your back, or shrug your shoulders.

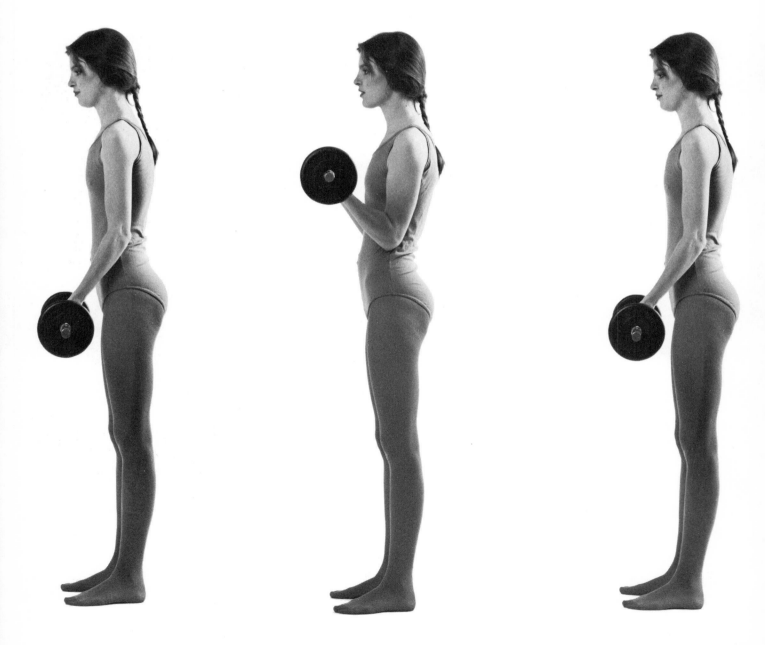

Arms

65. Lying Dumbbell Triceps Presses:
One set.
Fifteen repetitions with each arm.

This is for the triceps, the muscles at the back of your upper arms. As with the previous exercise, you must do it strictly to get much benefit from it.

Lie on the bench, on your back, your right leg bent with the foot on the bench, and your right arm extended over you, holding a dumbbell. (I like to keep my left hand on my right triceps to make sure the muscle is moving properly.) Bending your arm at the elbow, lower the dumbbell to your ear, then raise it again for one rep. Make sure that your upper arm doesn't move and that your elbow remains pointed directly at the ceiling through each rep. Do fifteen with the right arm, then fifteen with the left.

Program Five

(Intermediate)
Target Time:
Thirty-one minutes

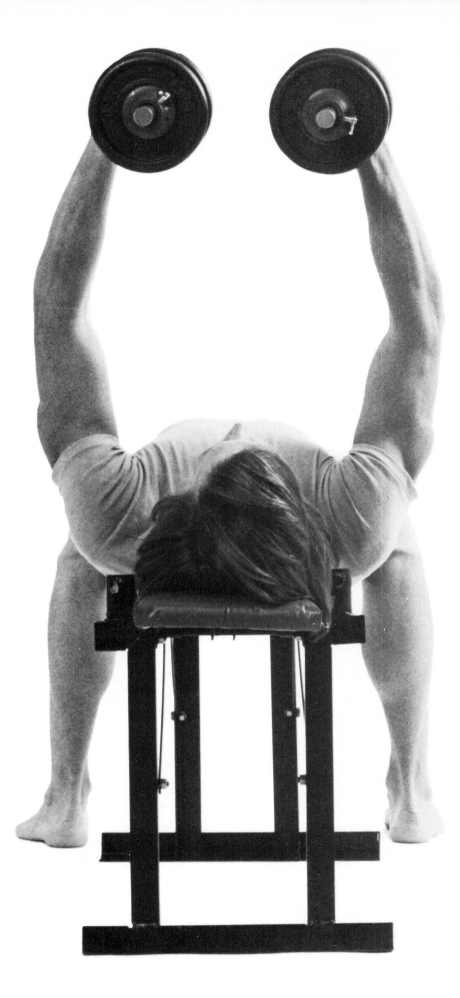

Waist

66. Sit-ups:
One set.
Fifty repetitions.

This is an excellent waist-hardening sit-up, good for your back too.

Sit with your legs bent and your feet underneath something solid. Put your hands on the small of your back, right at your belt-line, with the palms facing out. Drop back until your palms touch the floor, then sit up again for one rep.

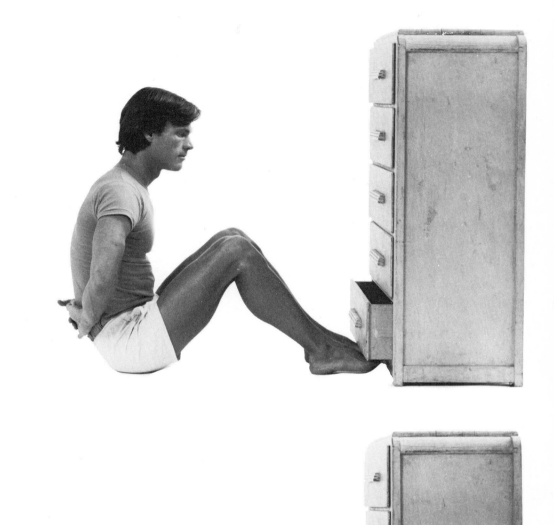

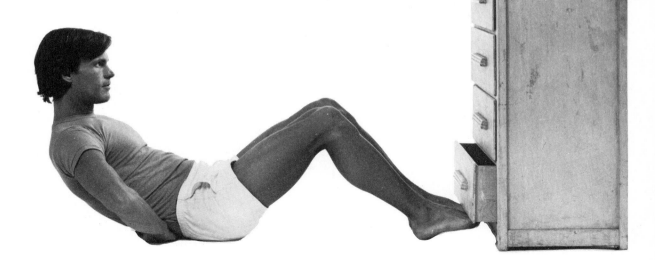

Waist

67. Leg Raises:
One set.
Fifteen repetitions.

To do this exercise for the lower abdominals, lie on your back with your hands underneath your buttocks and your legs together. Keeping your legs straight, lift them six inches off the floor and hold them there for a count of three, for one repetition.

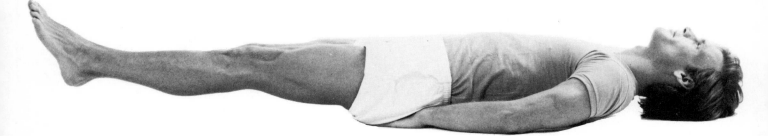

Waist

68. Side Bends with Dumbbell:
One set.
Twenty repetitions.

This exercise is for the soft-tending oblique muscles at the sides of your waist.

Stand with your feet about a foot apart, holding a dumbbell in each hand at your sides. Bending only sideways, dip to the right until the dumbbell comes near the side of your knee. Now come back up, and without stopping at the vertical bend to the other side for one repetition. Do these quickly.

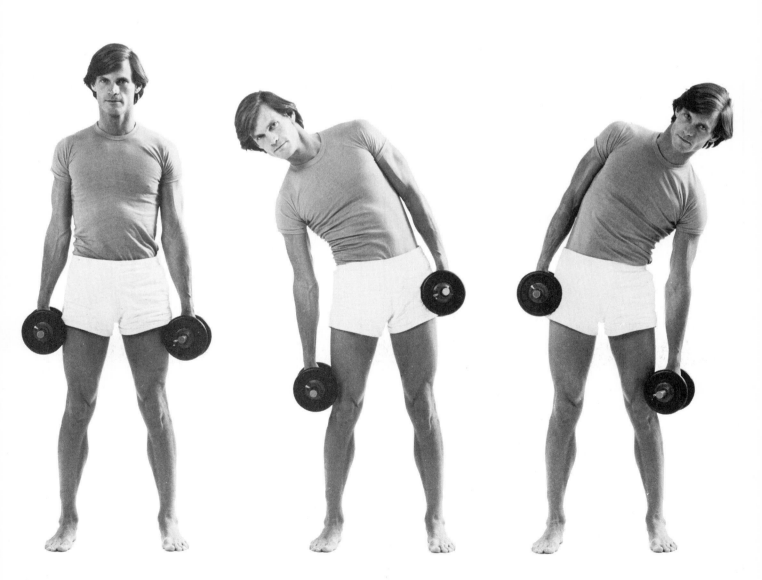

Waist

69. Standing Twists with Barbell:
One set.
Fifteen repetitions to each side.

These twists tone the upper and lower abdominals, the obliques, and the intercostals. They are also good for a sore lower back and for your flexibility.

Stand with your feet a little more than shoulder width apart, holding the barbell behind your neck on your shoulders in a wide grip. Without moving your feet, twist as far to the right as you can, letting your body from the knees to the head come around; then come back to the original position, for one repetition. Now do one to the left, and fourteen more to each side.

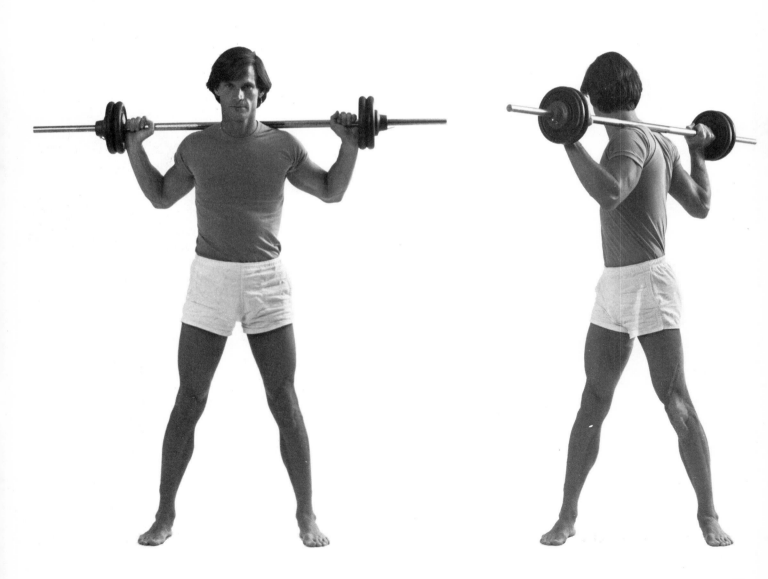

Legs and Buttocks

70. Alternating Standing Kick-backs:
One set.
Twenty-five repetitions with each leg.

This exercise tones your buttocks and hips. It is an excellent jogging warm-up, and massages your lower back.

Place your feet together two and a half to three feet away from a bench or stool. Bend over and put your hands on the bench, so that your head is only slightly higher than your hips. Now raise your right leg, with your foot turned sideways, until it makes a straight line with your back. Lower it and do the left. Alternate for twenty-five reps with each.

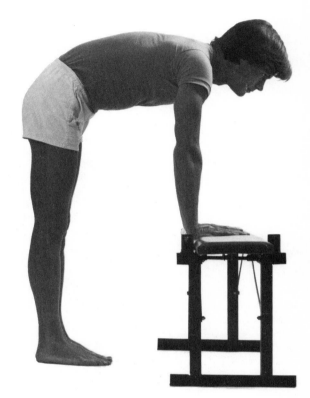

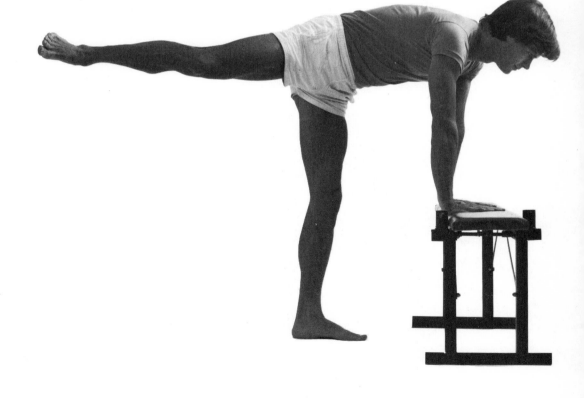

Legs and Buttocks

71. Knee Bends to Chair:
One set.
Fifteen repetitions.

This is for your upper legs and hips. Stand in front of a chair, your heels on a block, your feet a few inches apart, and holding two dumbbells at your sides. Holding your back very straight, sink down until your buttocks touch the chair and then stand back up for one rep. Your heels should remain on the block on the way up.

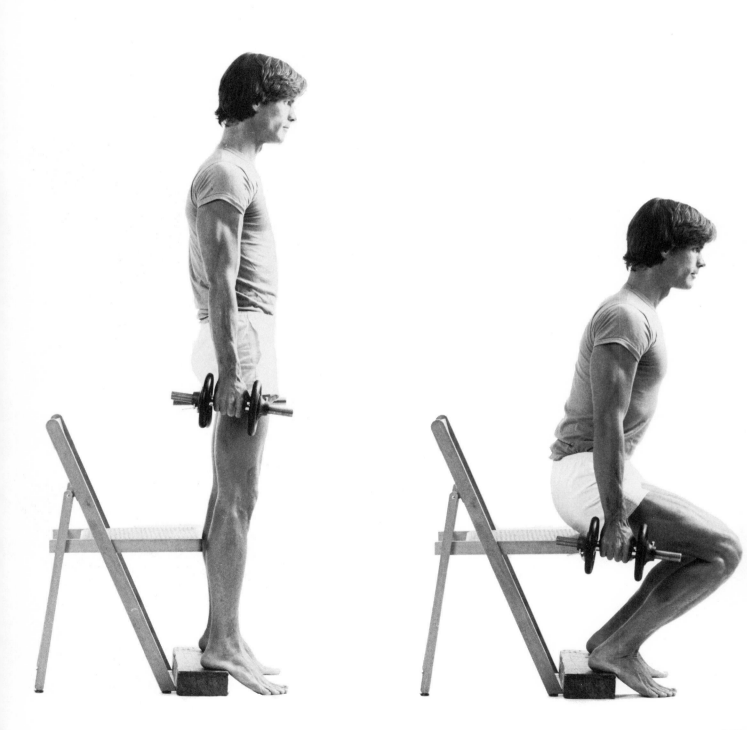

Legs and Buttocks

72. Lying Leg Curls:
One set.
Fifteen repetitions.

This exercise, for the biceps femoris at the back of your upper legs, relies considerably on concentration. Lie on the bench with your head lifted and your lower legs extending beyond one end. Hold onto the legs of the bench with your hands. Keeping your toes pointed toward the floor, curl your heels up toward your buttocks as far as they will come, imagining and feeling as you do it that your legs are weighted. Tense the hamstring muscles and force them to curl your heels upward against an imagined downward force.

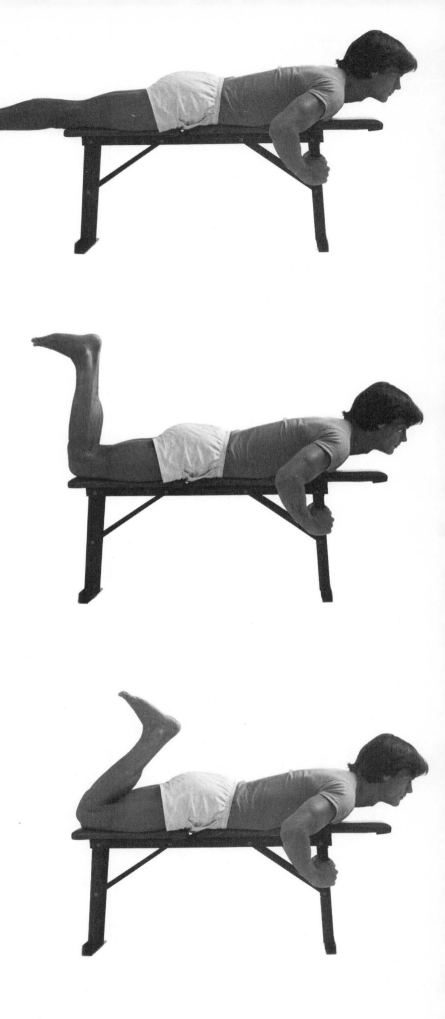

Legs and Buttocks

73. One-Leg Calf Raises:
One set.
Twenty repetitions with each leg.

Do this calf-toning exercise one leg at a time, holding a dumbbell on the same side as the leg being worked, and with the opposite hand holding onto something for balance. Stand with the ball of the foot on a ledge or block, the heel dangling as far down as you can push it. Now stand up as high as you can on your toes for one rep. Do twenty with each calf.

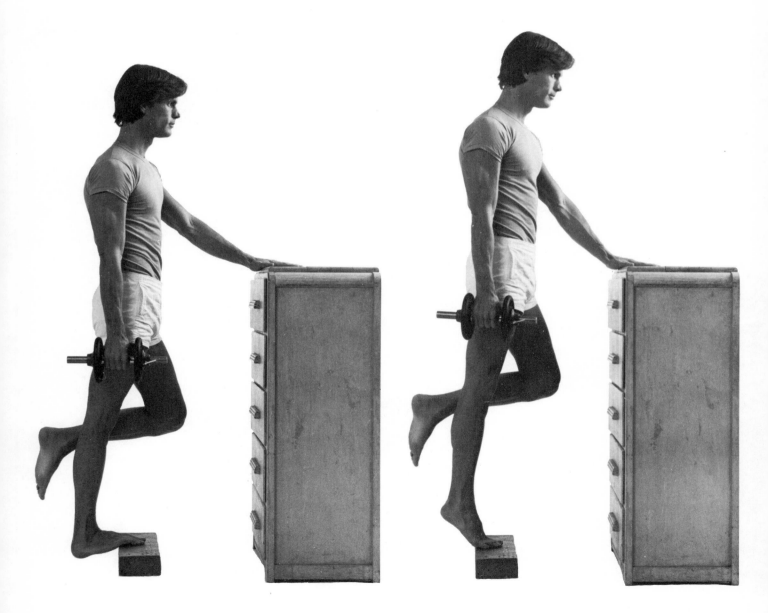

Chest

74. Bench Presses:
One set.
Twenty repetitions.

Probably the best exercise there is for the pectorals. To do them, lie on your back on the bench, your feet spread wide, holding the bar on your chest in as wide a grip as you can take between the weights. Raise the bar an inch or two off your chest and use that position as the bottom of each repetition in order to keep tension on the muscles.

Push the bar straight up, but don't lock out your elbows; lower it again smoothly for one repetition.

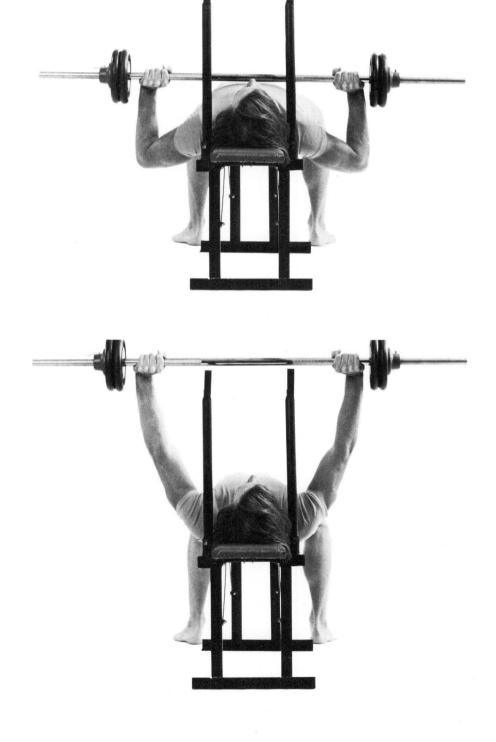

Chest

75. Dumbbell Flies:
One set.
Twenty repetitions.

This is an excellent overall chest exercise, and particularly good for women.

Take the same position on the bench as in the previous exercise, holding the two dumbbells over your chest, your arms bent slightly at the elbows. Keeping your arms bent, lower the weights to the level of the bench (your elbows should drop beneath it) and bring them smoothly back up, keeping tension on your chest. Don't quite let the dumbbells touch at the top of the rep.

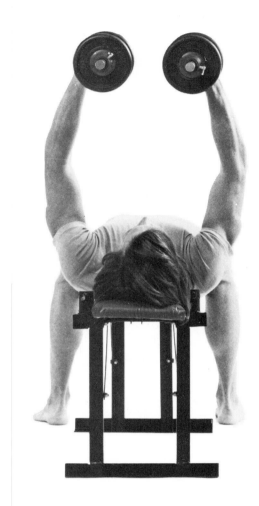

76. Alternating Dumbbell Rows:
One set.
Twenty repetitions with each arm.

This row works primarily on the latissimus
dorsi, but because of the position of the
body it also tones the teres and other muscles of the upper back.

Standing with your legs slightly bent at the
knees and holding both dumbbells, bend at
the waist and place your head on a chair or
something else at about knee level. The
dumbbells should be near but not quite
touching the floor. Relax your arms so that
the exercise can happen in your back. Now
lift the dumbbell in your right hand until it
touches your chest; then lower it, and lift the
one in your left hand. Alternate for twenty
repetitions with each arm.

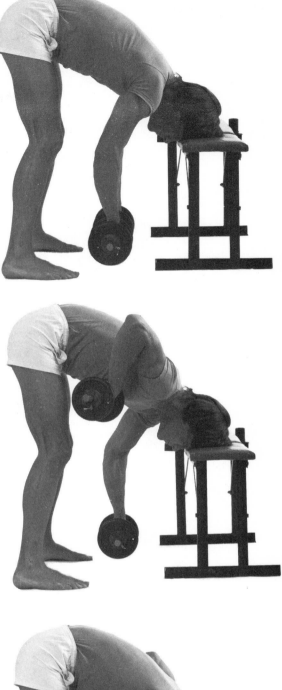

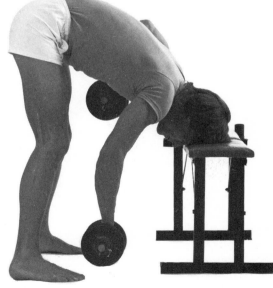

Back

77. Stand-ups with Barbell:
One set.
Fifteen repetitions.

This exercise tones the lower back, particularly the spinal erector muscles.

Place the barbell on the floor. With your feet shoulder width apart and about a foot away from the bar, bend over at the waist, legs straight, knees unbent, and take a wide grip on the bar. Now let your lower-back muscles pull you up into a perfectly erect position. Go back down slowly, again putting the tension on the back, for one repetition.

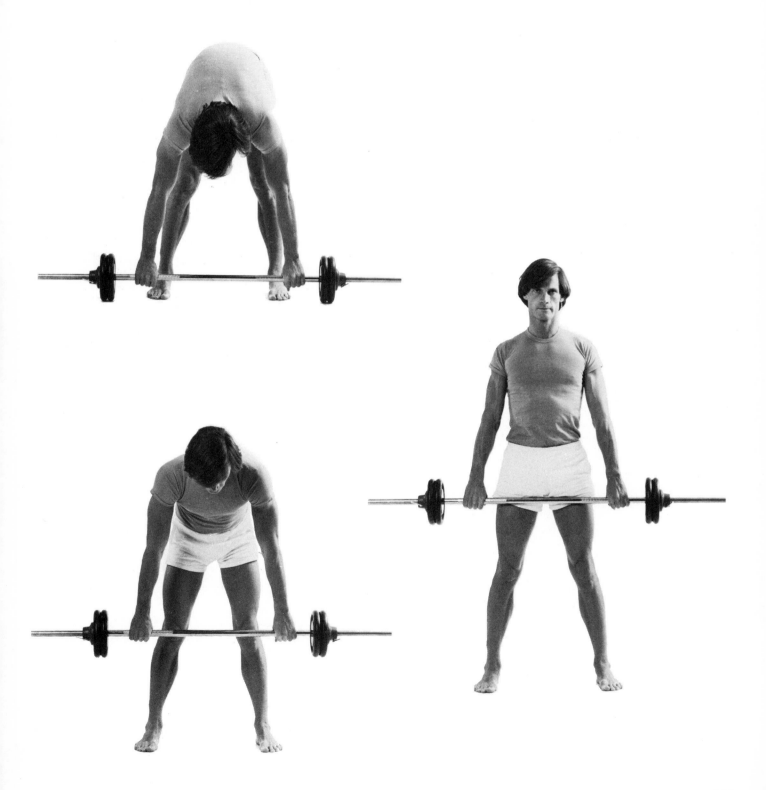

Shoulders

78. Standing Barbell Presses:
One set.
Twenty repetitions.

The press shown here tones all three heads of the deltoid muscles. If you have a bad lower back, be particularly careful to keep your back absolutely straight as you do the exercise.

Stand, feet shoulder width apart, holding the bar with a wide grip at the top of your chest. Press straight up, without bending your back or moving any part of your body but your arms, to full extension, then lower the bar smoothly, for one repetition.

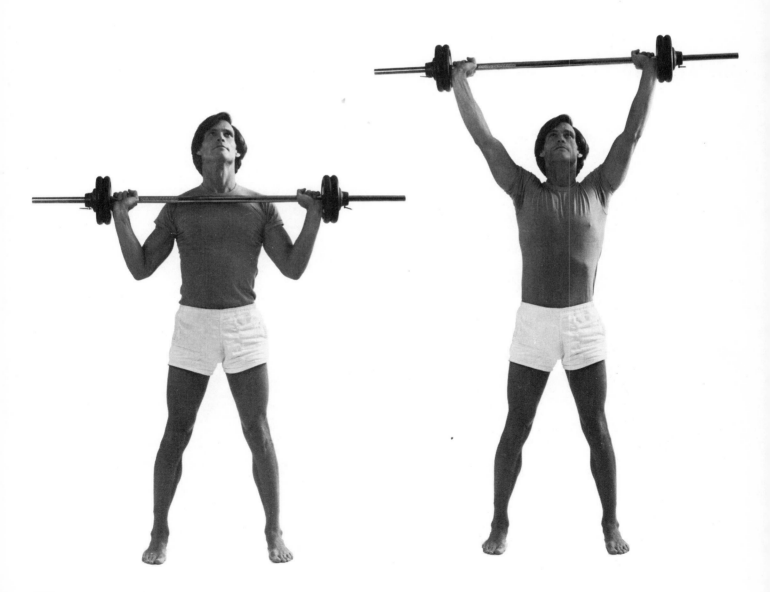

Shoulders

79. Front Raises with Barbell:
One set.
Fifteen repetitions.

This is an excellent shoulder conditioner, particularly for the frontal deltoid. Stand with feet twelve to eighteen inches apart, holding the bar near its center. Keeping your arms straight, raise the bar to eye level and hold for a count of two before lowering it, slowly, for one repetition.

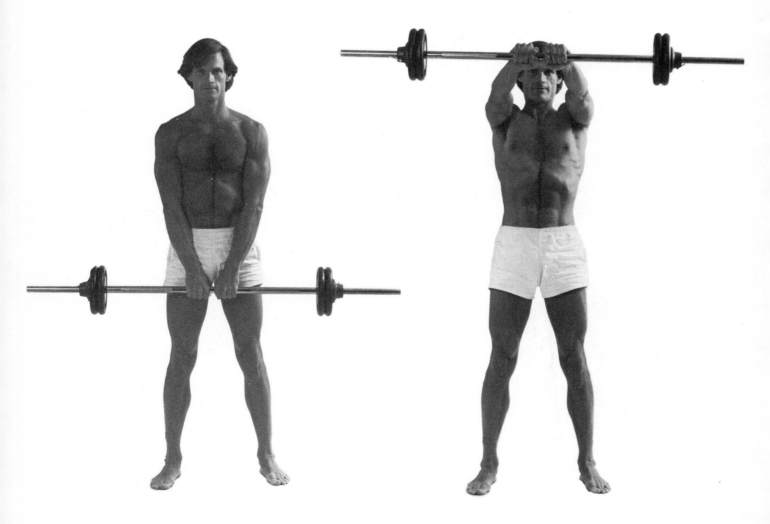

Arms

80. Seated Dumbbell Curls:
One set.
Twenty repetitions.

This exercise for toning the biceps is done seated in a chair, your back straight, your arms held out slightly from your sides, and your hands holding the dumbbells below your hips with the palms facing upward. Now, keeping the backs of your arms rigid and without moving your back, curl both dumbbells up toward your shoulders. Bring them only as high as there is still tension on the fronts of your upper arms, then lower them slowly, keeping the tension there, for one rep.

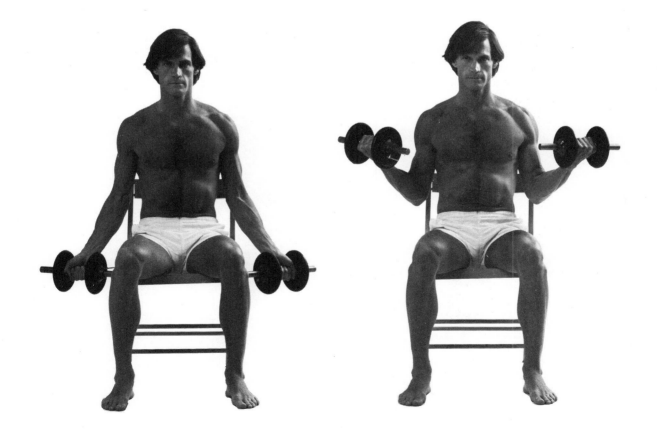

Arms

81. Seated Dumbbell Triceps Presses:
One set.
Fifteen repetitions with each arm.

This and the last exercise in this program are for hardening up the backs of your arms, and for the exercises to work properly you have to concentrate on that area.

Sit on a bench or in a chair, your back straight, holding a dumbbell overhead in your right hand. Using your elbow as a hinge, lower the dumbbell behind your head. Your elbow should be pointed directly at the ceiling and your upper arm shouldn't move. Now raise it again smoothly, keeping your upper arm steady, for one repetition. Do fifteen with your right arm, then fifteen with your left.

82. Triceps Extensions with Dumbbell:
One set.
Fifteen repetitions with each arm.

Stand a couple of feet away from a bench or a chair—something about knee level. Bend at the waist until your back is flat and put your left hand on the bench or chair. Hold the dumbbell in your right hand, close to your chest with your elbow bent. Now, without moving your shoulder or upper arm, extend the dumbbell backward until your arm is straight, then bring it back down slowly for one repetition.

Program Six

(Advanced)
Target Time:
Forty minutes

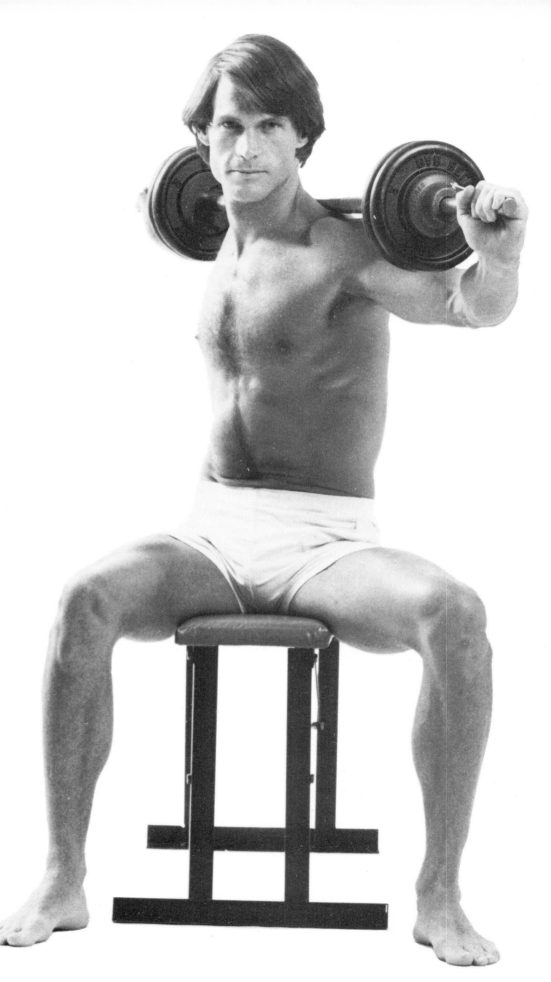

Waist

83. Sit-ups:
One set.
One hundred repetitions.

This sit-up is an excellent waist toner. It works both the upper and lower abdominals and is also good for limbering up a stiff lower back.

Sit with your feet under something immovable, your knees bent and your hands clasped behind your head. Go down until your lower back touches the floor, and then sit back up. Do repetitions smoothly and quickly.

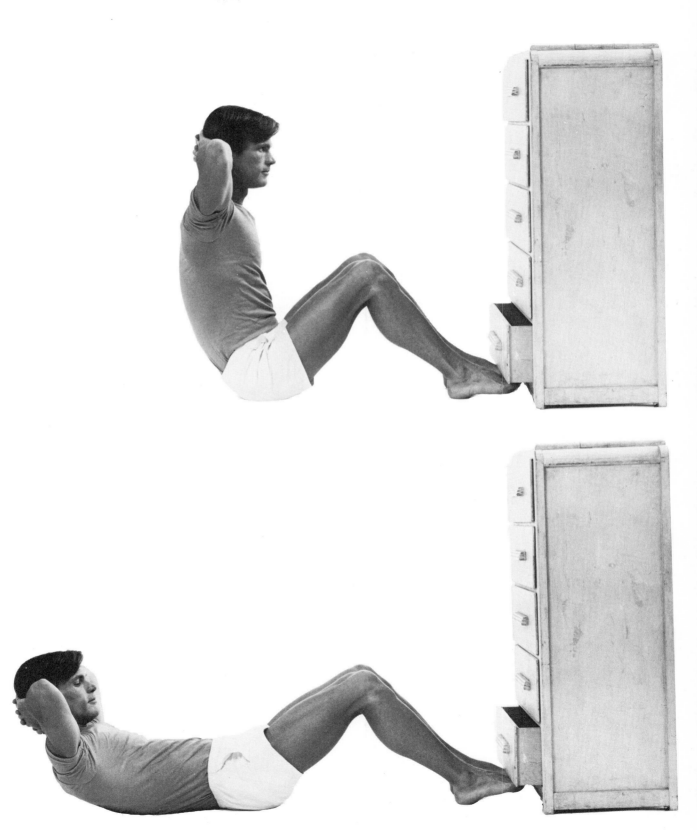

Waist

84. Seated Crunches:
One set.
Fifty repetitions.

This is another fine waist-hardening exercise —one that takes a little getting used to. Because of the dual movement, it works the entire front of the waist.

Sit on the bench balanced on your buttocks, with your legs lifted and slightly bent, your arms stretched out horizontally, and your back raised at the angle shown. Now pull your knees and chest in toward each other at the same time, tensing your stomach muscles as you do it, then stretch back out again for one repetition. Do these quickly and develop a rhythm for them.

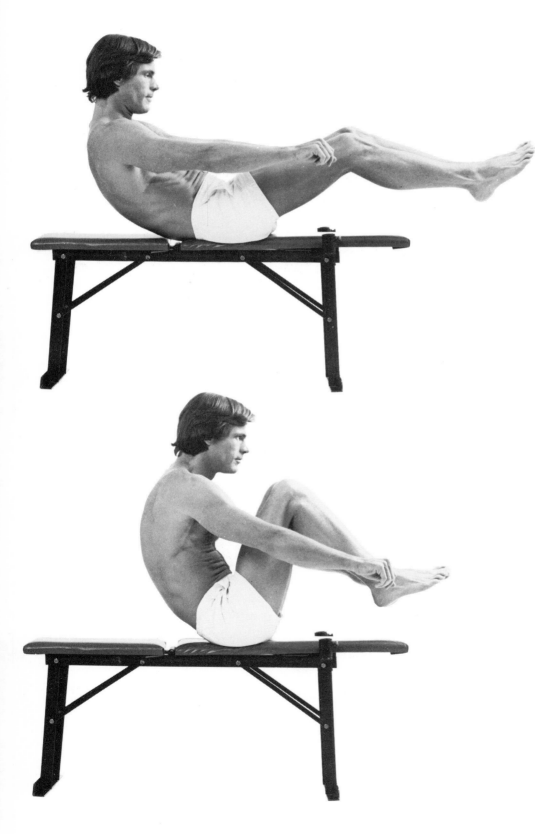

Waist

85. Side Bends with Dumbbell:
One set.
Twenty-five repetitions to each side.

For toning the oblique muscles along the sides of your waist and for tearing down fat tissue there.

Stand with your feet shoulder width apart, holding a dumbbell in your right hand. Keeping your back straight, bend to the right as far as you can and bring your left arm up over your head. Do twenty-five to that side, then put the dumbbell in your left hand and do twenty-five to the left. You should feel the exercise pulling the sides of your waist.

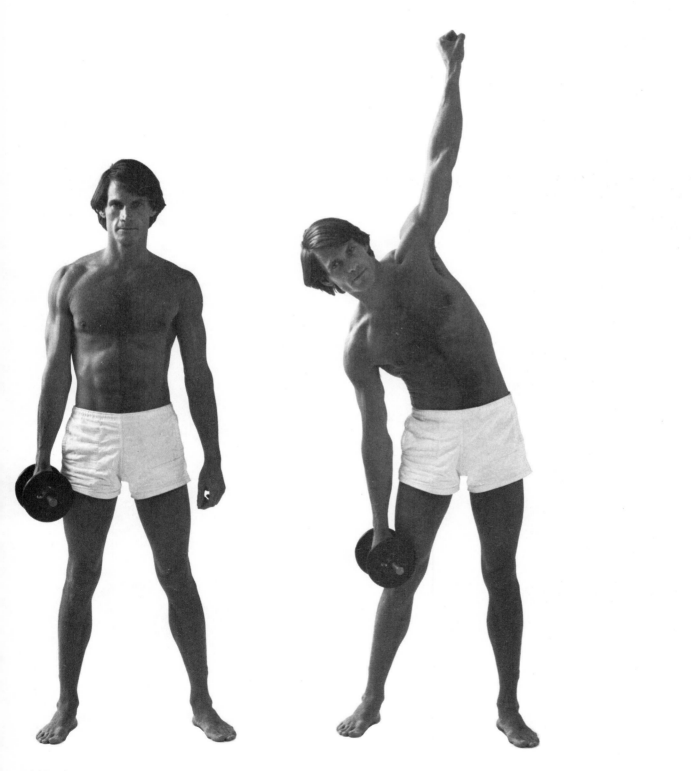

Waist

86. Seated Twists with Barbell:
One set.
Thirty-five repetitions to each side.

An all-around toner for the abdominals, the obliques, and the intercostals, this exercise should be done quickly but correctly.

Sit on the bench with the bar lying behind your neck and your hands as wide on it as possible. Twist at the waist as far as you can to the right without moving your head or hips. Come back to the first position for one rep, then twist in the other direction. Do thirty-five to each side.

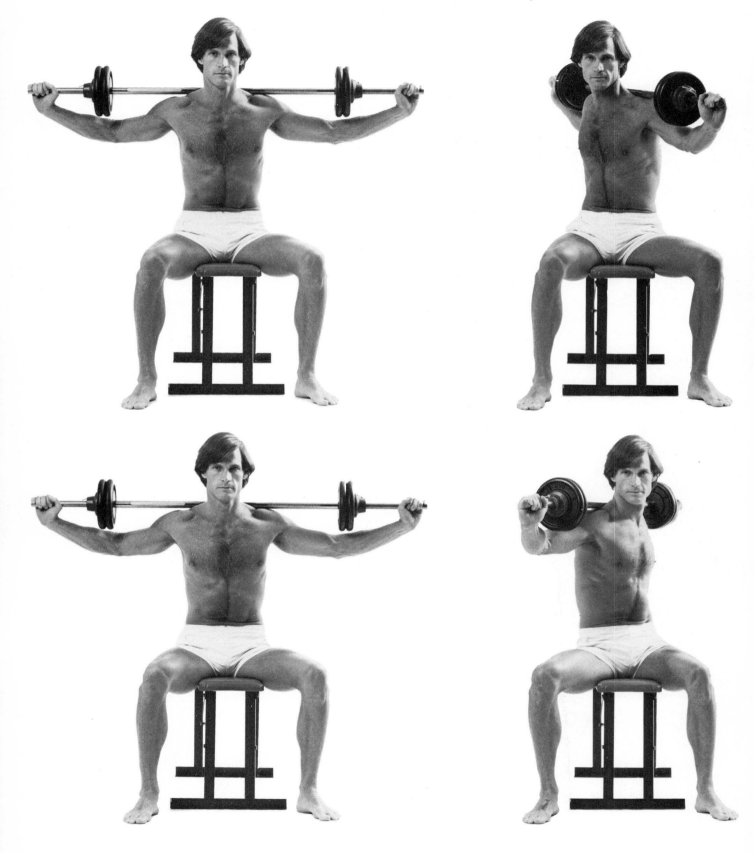

Waist

87. Standing Sweeps:
One set.
Fifteen repetitions in each direction.

This exercise tones all the muscles around the waist, strengthens your lower back, and is very good for torso flexibility. It is a good warm-up exercise for all sports.

Stand with your feet a little more than shoulder width apart, your hands on your hips and bent forward a little at the waist. Keep your head up. Now begin a circular sweeping motion to the right or left, stretching out fully to each side and at the back of the circle, and come back to the original position, for one repetition. Do fifteen in one direction, then reverse and do fifteen in the other.

Legs and Buttocks

88. Squats:
One set.
Thirty repetitions.

This is one of the best leg-toning exercises there is. It also reaches and tones muscles in the buttocks.

Stand with the bar on your shoulders and your heels elevated three to five inches on a book or a block of wood. Your feet should be about a foot apart. Keeping your back straight—not vertical, but flat—sink down to where your buttocks are at knee level or slightly below, then stand smoothly back up for one repetition. Your heels should remain flat on the block throughout.

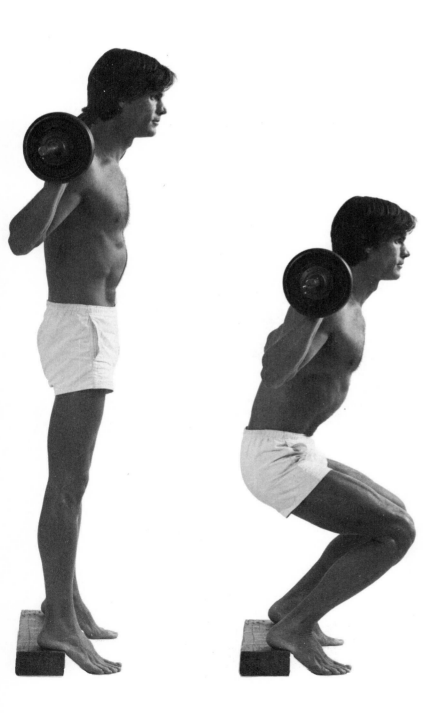

Legs and Buttocks

89. Lunges with Barbell:
One set.
Ten repetitions with each leg.

This is a wonderful exercise for your upper legs; it's also good for your balance, your flexibility, and your performance at a lot of sports, notably both kinds of skiing.

Stand with the bar on your shoulders and your hands wide on it. Step out with your right foot and sink down so that your left knee touches the floor; then push back up, using your right thigh muscles, and draw your feet together to the original position, for one repetition. Now lunge onto the left leg, and alternate for ten with each.

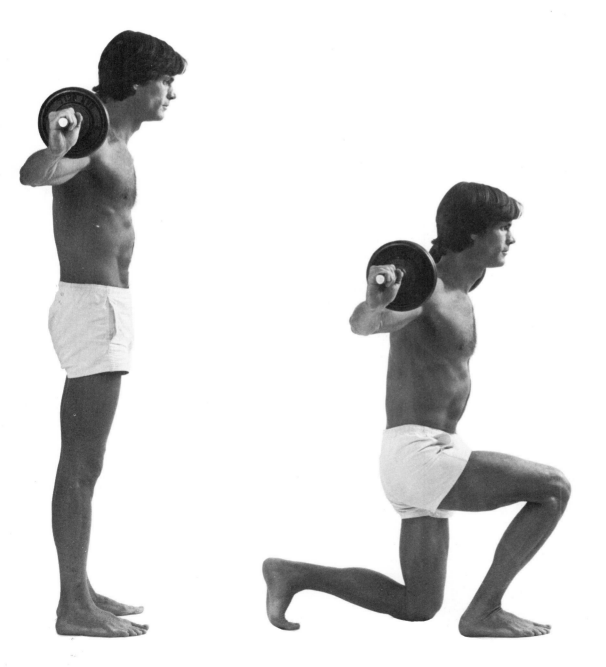

Legs and Buttocks

90. Leg Curls with Dumbbell:
One set.
Fifteen repetitions with each leg.

This is for toning the backs of the legs; to do it you will need a belt or a strap. Put one end of the strap around the dumbbell and the other end around the ankle of your right leg.

Bend at the waist so that your back is flat and hold onto something. Lift your right leg behind you so that the dumbbell is just off the floor (it should not touch the floor throughout the exercise). Now curl your heel up toward your buttocks as far as it will go and lower it again smoothly for one repetition. Do fifteen with the right leg, then fifteen with the left.

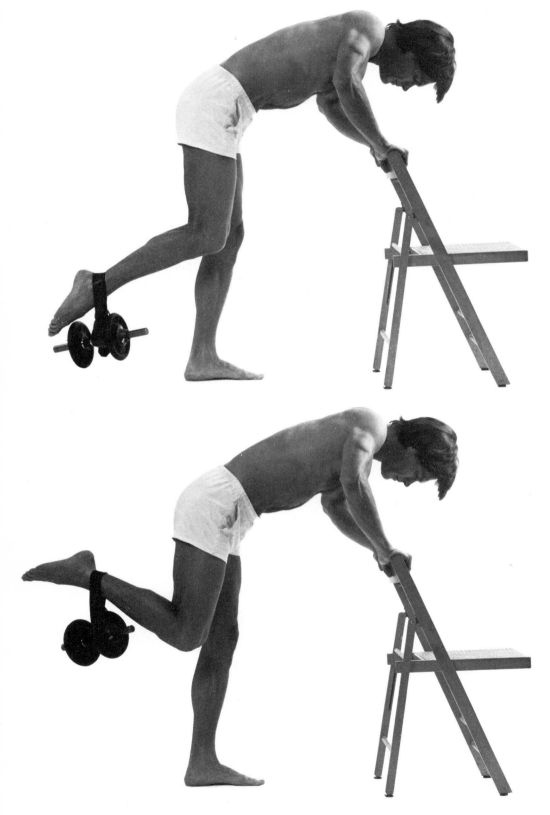

Legs and Buttocks

91. Calf Raises with Barbell:
One set.
Thirty repetitions.

For these calf-toning and -shaping raises, stand with your toes and the first inch or two of your insteps on a ledge or high block. Hold the barbell in a wide grip on your shoulders behind your neck. Go straight up on your toes as far as you can stretch, hold the rep at the top for a count of two, then come back down, letting your heels drop as far down as possible, for one repetition.

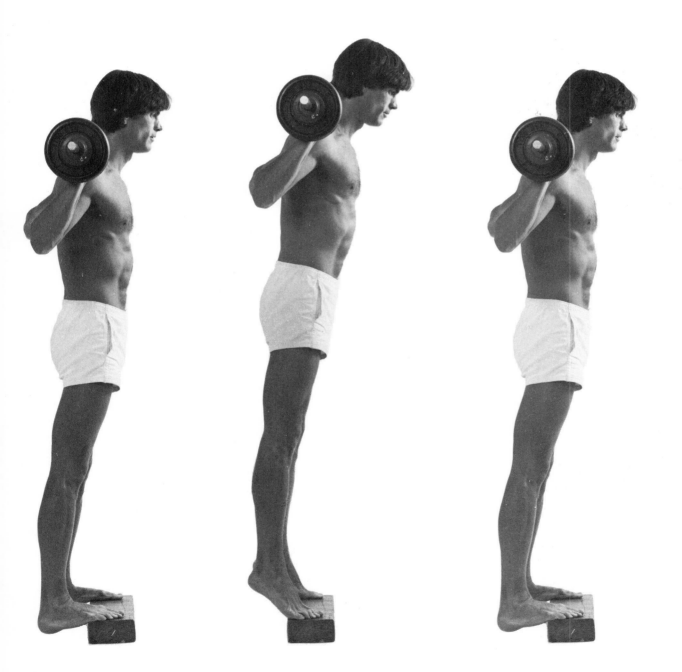

Chest

92. Benchpress Pull-overs:
One set.
Twenty repetitions.

This two-part exercise hardens the pectorals, the serratus muscles, the intercostals, and even the upper abdominals. Lie on your back on the bench with your feet up on one end and your head just off the other. Start with the bar on your chest, held with your hands inside your shoulders. Press the bar over your chest to full arm extension, lower it again to an inch or two above your chest, then push it out, over and behind your head, until it touches the floor. For the last movement of the exercise, bring the bar smoothly back up—using your chest muscles to pull it—to the original position, for one repetition.

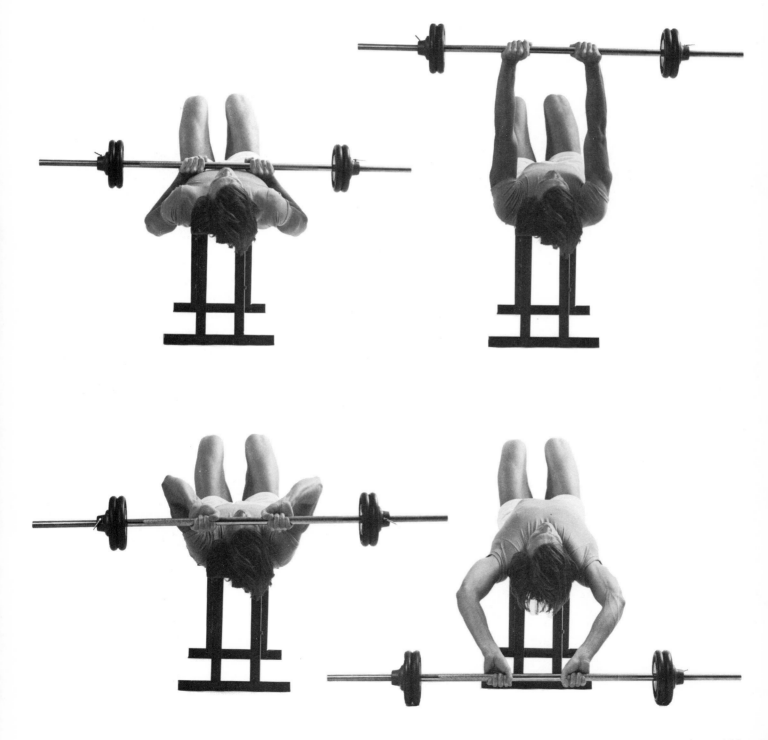

Chest

93. Standing Dumbbell Flies:
One set.
Twenty repetitions.

This is a superb chest hardener. Stand with your feet close together, holding the two dumbbells out to your sides, your arms fully extended, the bars of the dumbbells parallel to the floor. Without arching your back, bring the dumbbells in toward each other and keep them going across your body until your right arm crosses your left at the elbows. On the next rep, cross the left arm over the right, and continue alternating for twenty repetitions.

Some of you women may find it impossible to cross your arms with the weights; if so, just bring the dumbbells together in front of you at neck level.

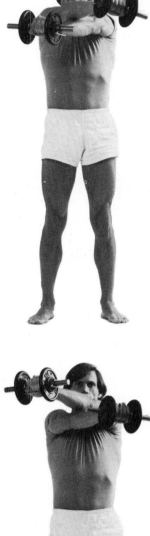

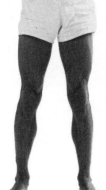

Back

94. Barbell Rows:
One set.
Twenty-five repetitions.

This exercise for toning the upper back is best done by standing on the bench, though it can also be done on the floor. With your feet together and your legs straight, bend forward at the waist with the barbell until it is an inch or two off the bench (it should not touch the bench throughout). Locate the strain of holding it in your back rather than your arms, then lift it until the bar touches your chest. Don't jerk the bar. Keep your back flat. Smoothly lower the bar for one repetition. You have to feel this exercise into the back muscles.

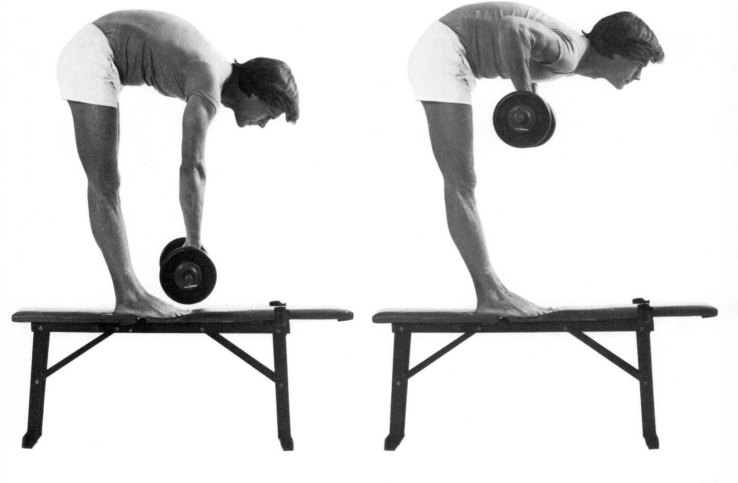

Back

94A. Alternate Exercise: Behind-the-Neck Chins:
One set.
Ten repetitions.

Those of you who are super-hard might want to do this alternative upper-back exercise. Find a stairwell, or tree limb, or beam—something you can chin yourself on. Take hold of it with your palms facing away from you, your hands about three feet apart. Now lift your feet off the ground and bend your knees. Pull yourself straight up until the thing you are chinning on touches the back of your neck. Now lower yourself slowly, for one repetition.

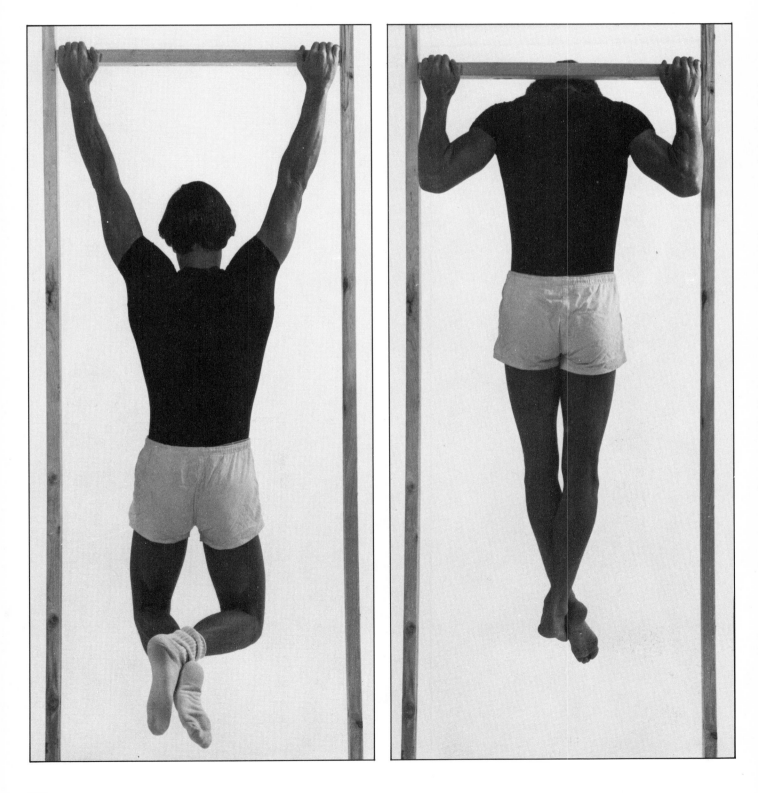

Back

95. Dumbbell Swings:
One set.
Twenty-five repetitions.

This hardens the lower back particularly, but is also good for the upper waist and the shoulders.

With your feet spaced a little wider than your shoulders, hold one or both dumbbells, depending on your strength, above your head. Swing your arms down between your legs, keeping your legs straight, and then back up without bending them much at the elbows. Make your lower back lift your body and arms back up to vertical.

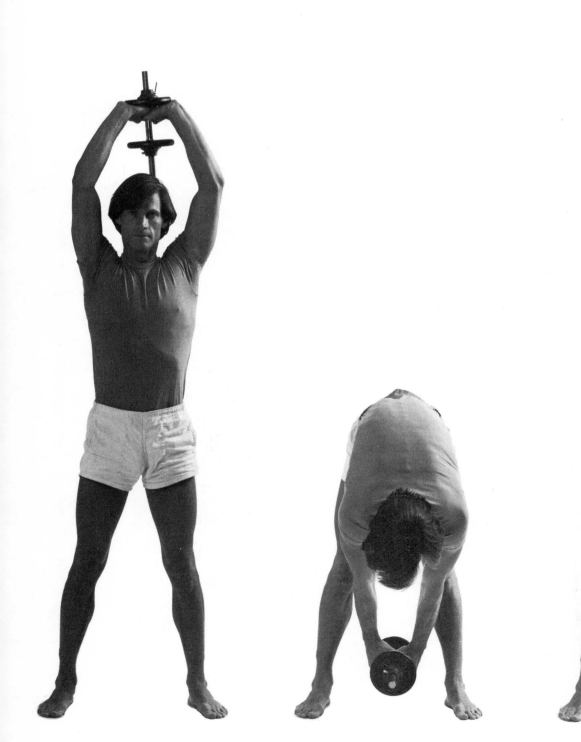

Shoulders

96. Seated Behind-the-Neck Presses with Barbell:
One set.
Twenty-five repetitions.

This exercise is for toning the deltoid muscles of the shoulder, particularly their rear heads, which tend to go soft the quickest.

Sit on the bench holding the bar behind your neck on your shoulders, your hands just wider than your shoulders. Lift the bar an inch or two off your shoulders and let this be the bottom position for each rep. Now press the barbell overhead, keeping your back straight, to an extension just short of locking your elbows. Lower slowly for one repetition.

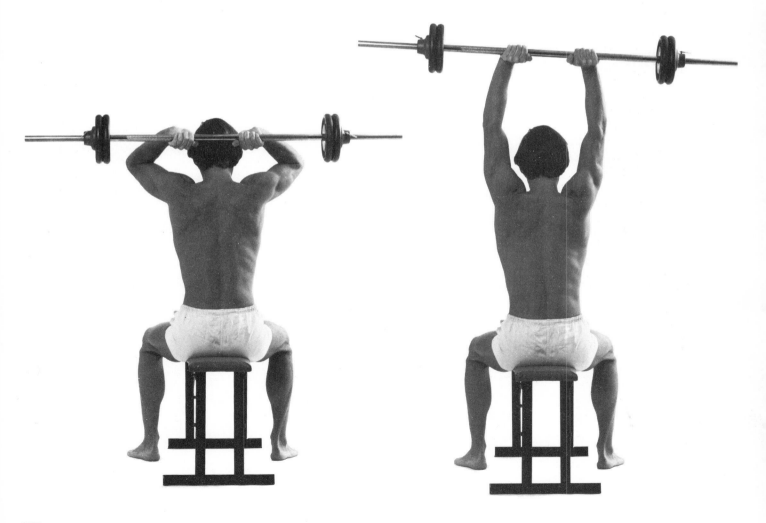

Shoulders

97. Standing Dumbbell Flies:
One set.
Twenty-five repetitions.

This is an overall shoulder toner, and it reaches the upper pectorals as well. Very few people do this exercise correctly; Arnold Schwarzenegger taught me how.

Stand with your feet shoulder width apart, holding the two dumbbells in front of your hips, palms facing each other, with your arms bent a little at the elbow, and leaning slightly forward at the waist. Now bring your arms up in front of your body, with the front end of each dumbbell tipped a little toward the floor as if you were pouring water out of it. Bring the dumbbells up just above your head and lower them to original position again smoothly for one repetition.

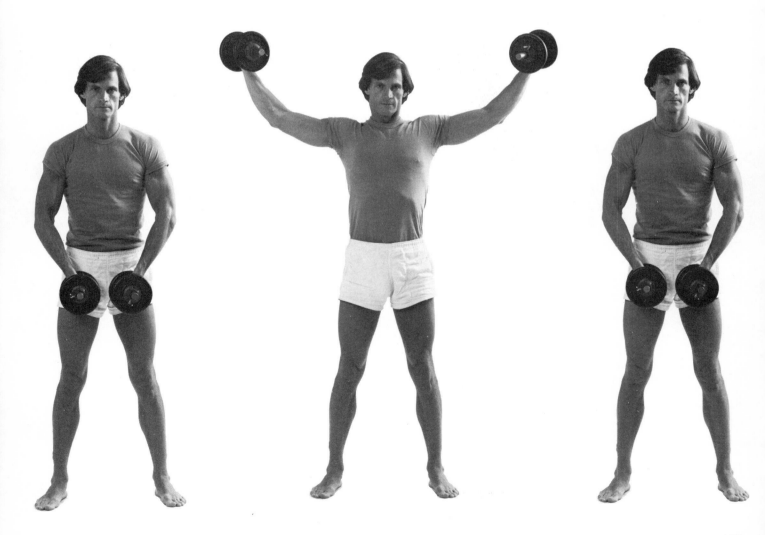

Arms

98. Barbell Curls on Back of Chair:
One set.
Twenty-five repetitions.

Kneel in or straddle a chair and hold the barbell over its back with your hands six to twelve inches apart. Lift the bar an inch or two, to where tension is placed on the biceps at the front of your upper arms. Keeping your body still, curl the bar up toward your chin as far as there is still tension on your arms. Don't swing the bar up, and let it back down slowly for the completion of the repetition. Concentrate the exercise into the biceps all the way through each rep.

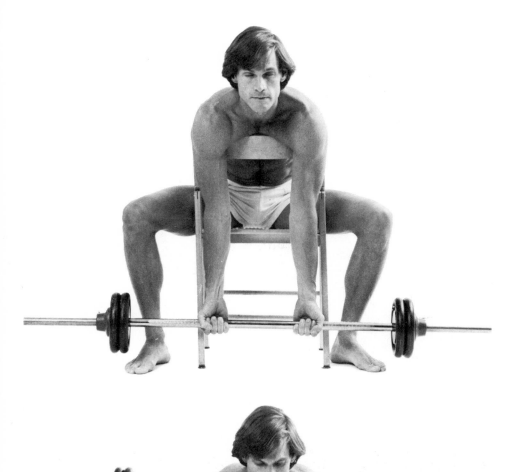

Arms

99. Lying Triceps Presses with Barbell:
One set.
Twenty-five repetitions.

This and the next exercise are both for toning the backs of your arms. The triceps muscle there has three parts, or heads, and this exercise is particularly good for the outside head.

Lie on your back on the bench. Hold the bar above your neck with your elbows locked and your hands only four or five inches apart. The bar should actually rest on the pads at the base of your fingers, not in your palms. Now, hinging at the elbows, leaving your upper arm absolutely still and the elbows pointed at the ceiling, slowly lower the bar to just behind your head so that the backs of your hands touch your scalp; then push the bar straight up again to your first position, making the backs of your arms do the work, for one repetition.

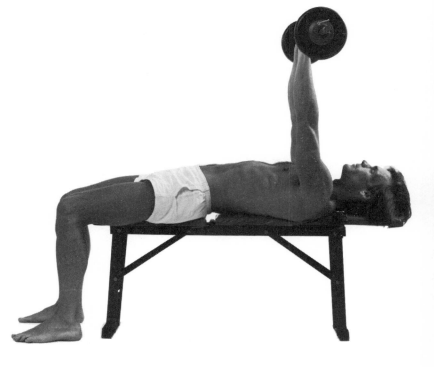

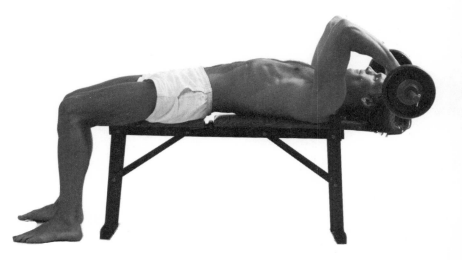

100. Seated Triceps Presses with Barbell:

One set.
Twenty-five repetitions.

This final exercise is a seated version of the last one, but because of the position of the arms, it reaches the inside and middle heads of the triceps better.

Sit on the bench with your back straight, holding the barbell overhead with your hands six inches apart. Hinging at the elbows in the same way described in the last exercise, lower the bar behind your neck as far as you can. Keep your upper arms still, elbows pointed up. Now, smoothly, using the backs of your arms, push the bar back up to overhead. Concentrate on the upward movement.

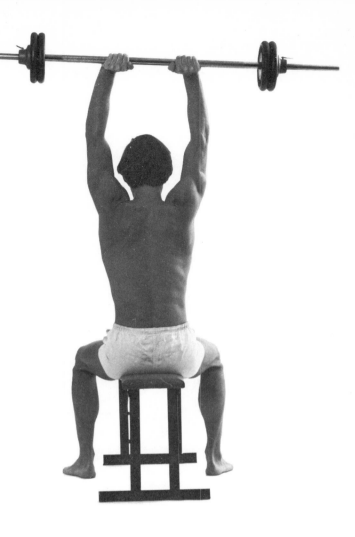

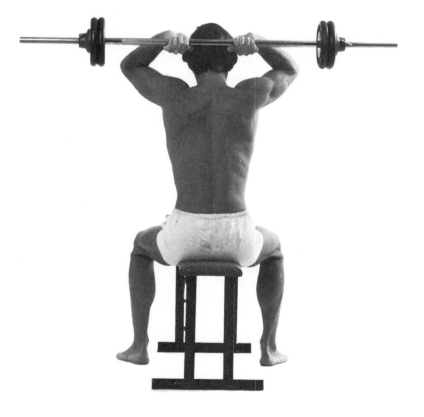

Section III:
Exercises on Universal Machines

To my mind the Universal multi-station machines are the best exercise machines available, and the best thing to happen for those who want to stay hard conveniently and on a limited amount of training time since the invention of the push-up. These machines are in gyms all over the place, and you can locate one in almost any city or town in the country. If you have easy access to one on a regular basis, and want a simple, fast, contained program for staying hard, this might be your section.

Anyone can use a Universal productively, and it seems to be a particularly good toning method for women. My wife and a group of her friends have been staying hard nicely on one for a couple of years. It is their favorite form of programmed exercise. One reason for that is that you can reach and tone every major muscle in the body with a Universal and, because of the way the thing is designed, do so with an almost limitless variety of exercises. I have used the machines off and on for fifteen years, and the exercises shown in this section represent just the best of the ones I have found that are good for toning.

As in the other two sections, the exercises in each program here are tested parts of an individual whole, not just exercises thrown together arbitrarily. So for best results, do the exercises in the sequences shown, and do them according to the directions. Remember to breathe correctly: Inhale on the relaxation phase of each exercise movement and exhale on the resistance phase.

The point here, as in Section II, is not to do these exercises with as much weight as possible, but to find an amount of weight for each that reaches and tones the worked muscles without rebuilding them larger. There is no formula that I know of to do that with a Universal machine like the one I suggested for the section on exercises with weights. To find the amount of weight you should use for each exercise in this section you have to experiment, exercise by exercise. Pick the program you think is right for you and experiment with each exercise until you find a poundage that burns but doesn't exhaust the muscles. The range of weight at some of the Universal stations goes from ten to over three hundred pounds. Don't let this confuse or scare you. You will be able to sense very quickly more or less where you belong in that range, and then it's just fine-tuning. After you have established your weight for each exercise, do the entire program to find out how close you are to the Target Time.

Once you are doing Program Nine within its Target Time using poundages that are right for you, you can add reps or weight for some or all the exercises if you like, but for staying hard there is no need to.

Program Seven

(Beginner)
Target Time:
Eighteen minutes

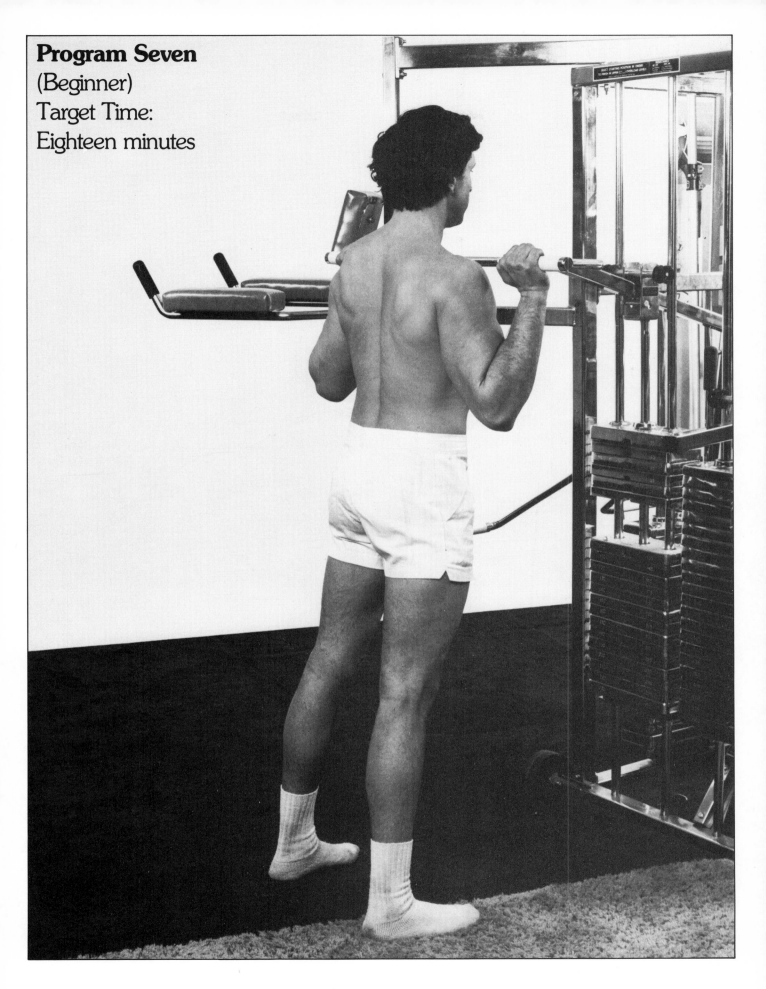

Waist

101. Sit-ups:
One set.
Twenty repetitions.

This particular sit-up tones both the upper and lower abdominals well. Its effectiveness is in direct proportion to how strictly you do it.

Lie on the slantboard, with the board flat on the floor, your feet hooked under the padded footholds, and your arms stretched out behind your head. Throw your arms up and forward, sit up behind them, and touch your toes; now go back smoothly to your original position. The more you pull yourself up with your stomach muscles, rather than throwing your body up with your arms, the more effective this sit-up becomes.

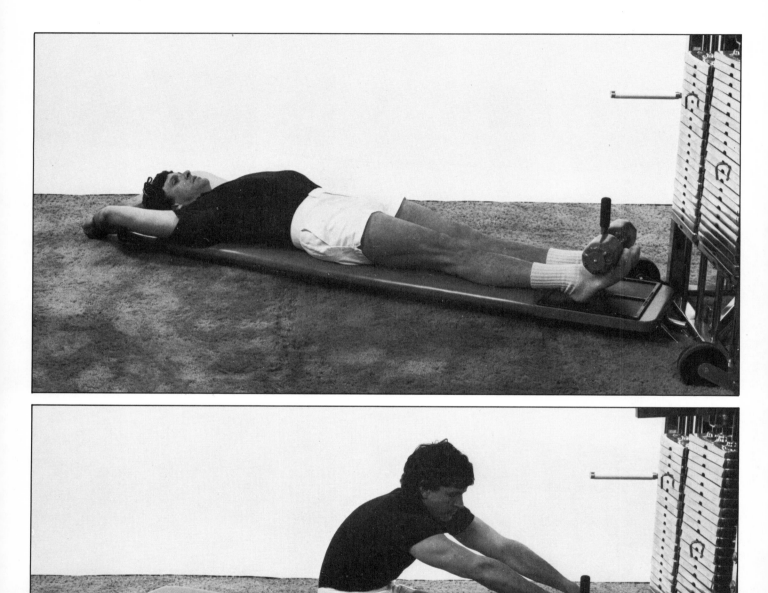

Waist

102. Leg Raises:
One set.
Fifteen repetitions.

This exercise works primarily on your lower abdominals, where soft tends to accumulate quickly. It is also good for lower-back problems and spinal flexibility.

Place the slantboard flat on the floor. Lie on it on your back with your head at the machine end and your hands holding the post. Keeping your legs as straight as possible, raise them until your feet are directly over your face, then lower them smoothly for one repetition.

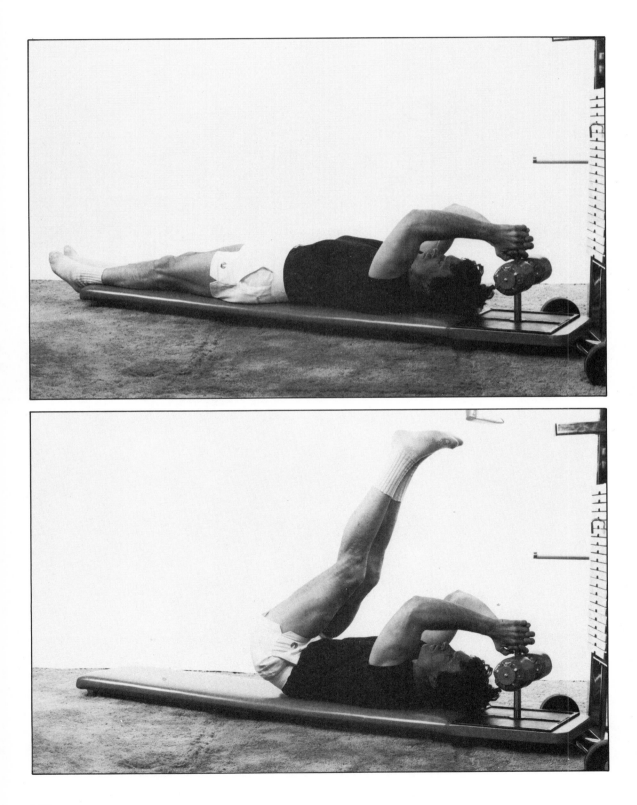

Waist

103. Sweeps:
One set.
Ten repetitions to each side.

Sweeps are an excellent warm-up exercise for all sports and a fine flexibility conditioner. They harden the abdominals, obliques, and intercostals. They are also a good hangover exercise.

Start in a standing position, your hands clasped over your head, and bent slightly backwards at the waist—enough so that your stomach muscles are tensed. Now sweep to the side in either direction—keeping your arms extended, describing a circle

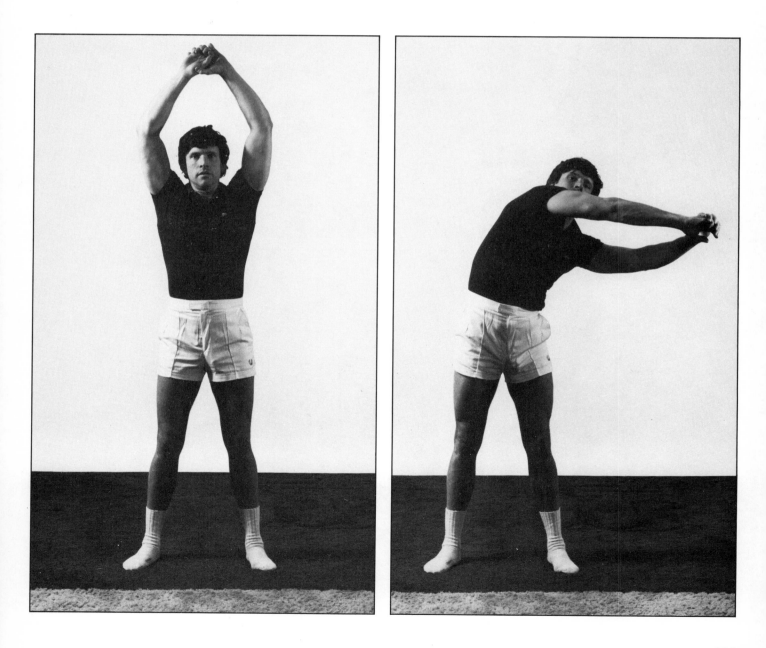

with them and your torso, and putting the strain of the exercise on the waist—all the way around and back to the original position for one repetition to that side. Do ten; then reverse the sweep and do ten in the other direction.

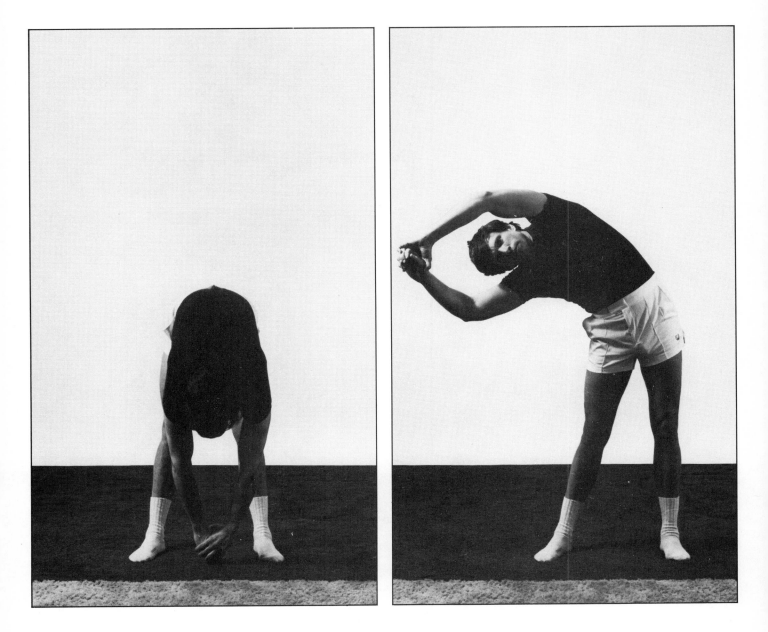

Legs and Buttocks

104. Flutter Kicks:
One set.
Twenty repetitions with each leg.

These kicks tone the back of the upper thighs and, particularly, the thighs and buttocks. They too are very good for your flexibility.

Lie with your stomach on the padded hyperextension platform, holding the chrome bar that runs beneath it. Now alternately kick each leg up and down, stretching as high as you can on the up motion.

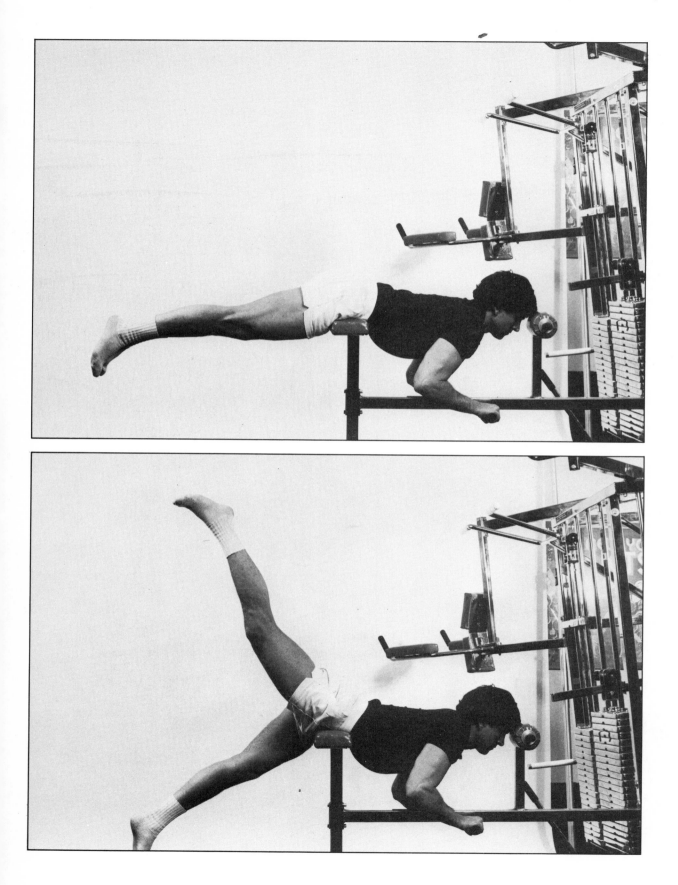

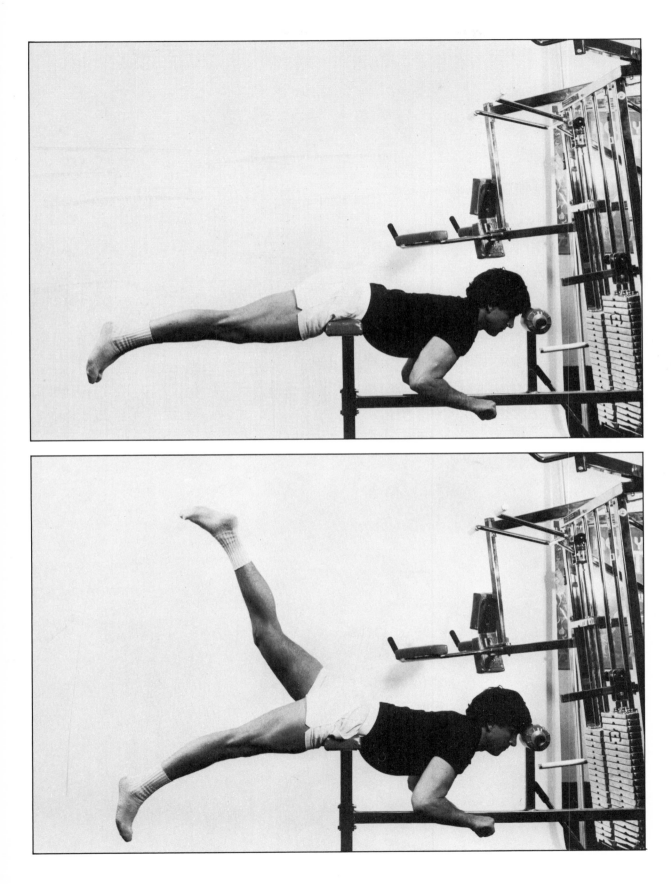

Legs and Buttocks

105. Leg Presses:
One set.
Fifteen repetitions.

This exercise is principally for toning the quadriceps—the four large muscles of your frontal thighs. It's a very good exercise for skiing, and other sports as well.

Pull the seat of the leg-press station (shown here) back to its outermost position. Sit holding your back flat against the back of the seat and place your feet on the bottom two metal rests. Without moving your upper body, push straight ahead until your legs are almost but not quite fully extended, then come slowly back to your original position for one repetition. Concentrate on these; feel your thigh muscles working.

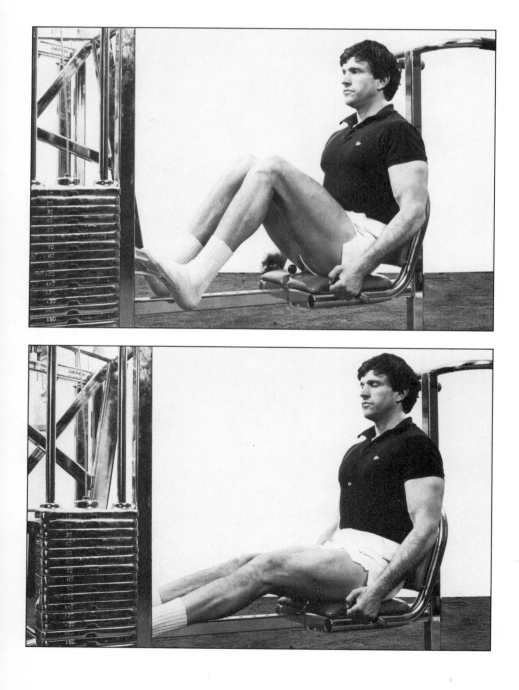

Legs and Buttocks

106. Calf Raises:
One set.
Fifteen repetitions.

For toning and shaping the calves, this exercise is done at the shoulder-press station of the machine. Get a block of wood four to six inches high and stand on it with your toes and the first inch or two of your instep, letting your heels hang off the back. Stand with your hands on the pressing bar, as close to it as you can get, with the station connected to at least thirty pounds. Without moving your hands, your back straight, stand up on your tiptoes, carrying the weight up as you go. Hold at the top for a count of two, then come back down to the original position. If you are doing this exercise correctly you will feel it only in your calves.

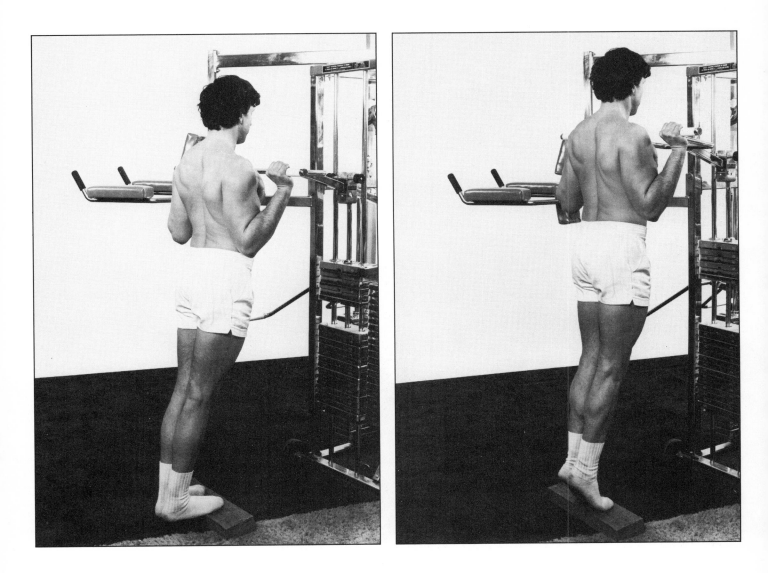

Chest

107. Bench Presses:
One set.
Fifteen repetitions.

Bench presses tone the pectoral muscles of the chest primarily, and are good for firming up a woman's breasts.

Lie flat-backed on the bench, your feet on the floor, holding the bars toward the outsides of the grips and so that your hands are at shoulder level. Push straight up to full extension of your arms. Let the weight back down smoothly and don't quite let it touch the plates below it—keeping tension on the chest—for one repetition.

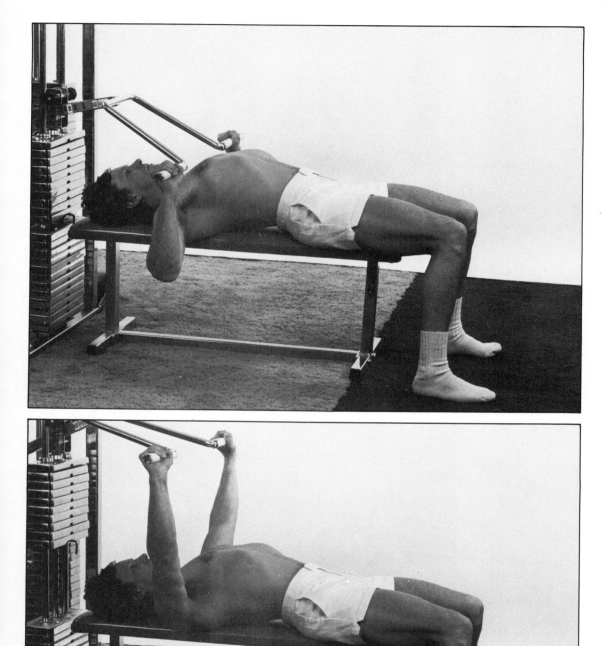

Chest

108. Pull-downs:
One set.
Fifteen repetitions.

This exercise for the pectoral and serratus muscles requires a good bit of concentration but is a wonderful hardener of the chest and rib-cage area.

Stand with your feet spread two to three feet apart, about a foot back from the dorsibar and pulley station shown here. Place your hands on the bar just on either side of the cable. Your arms should be only slightly bent. Now, keeping your back straight, pull the bar down toward your feet, using primarily your *chest* muscles—not your back, shoulders, or arms—to do it. Concentrate the exercise into your chest and you will feel it there.

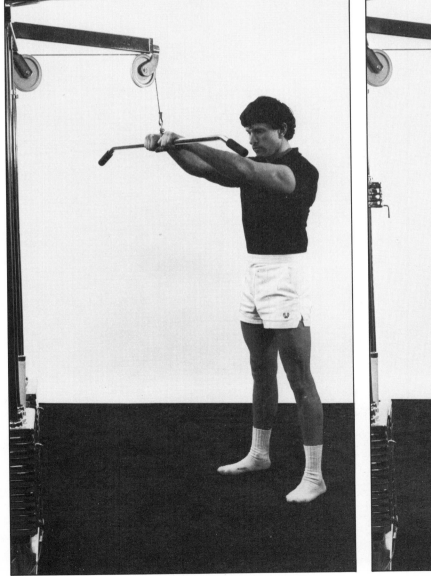
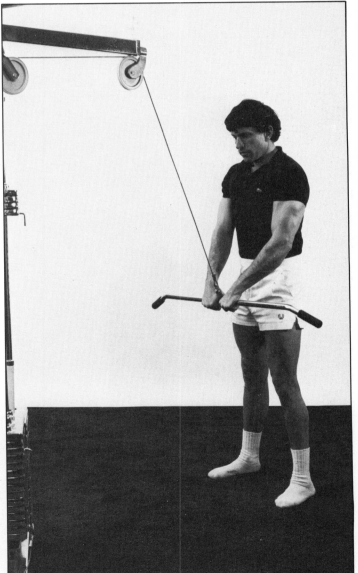

Back

109. Alms:
One set.
Fifteen repetitions.

This exercise looks much like the last one but, instead of the chest and rib cage, it reaches the latissimus dorsi muscles of the back when done correctly—the muscles from which this dorsi-bar station takes its name.

Kneel about a foot back from the bar, holding it overhead with your hands close together. Now pull the bar down with your arms straight until it comes below your waist, making a motion like the Eastern form of begging for which the exercise is named. Let the bar back up slowly to the original position for one repetition. You should feel this exercise along the sides of your back.

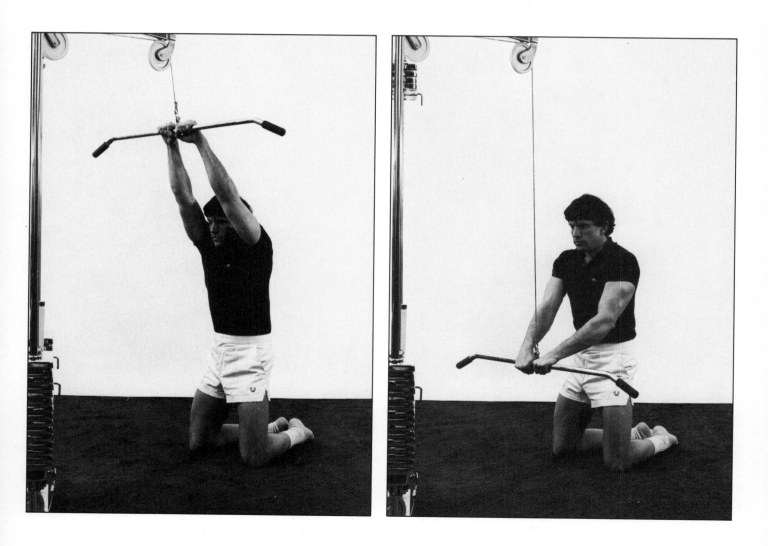

Back

110. Lat Pull-downs:
One set.
Fifteen repetitions.

This exercise, also for the latissimus dorsi, or lats, as well as other muscles in the back, is done like the previous two at the dorsi-bar station but probably with a bit more weight.

Again take a kneeling position, this time with your hands on the bar's grips and your body directly underneath it. Pull the bar smoothly down behind your neck, touching the backs of your shoulders, and let it smoothly back up for one repetition.

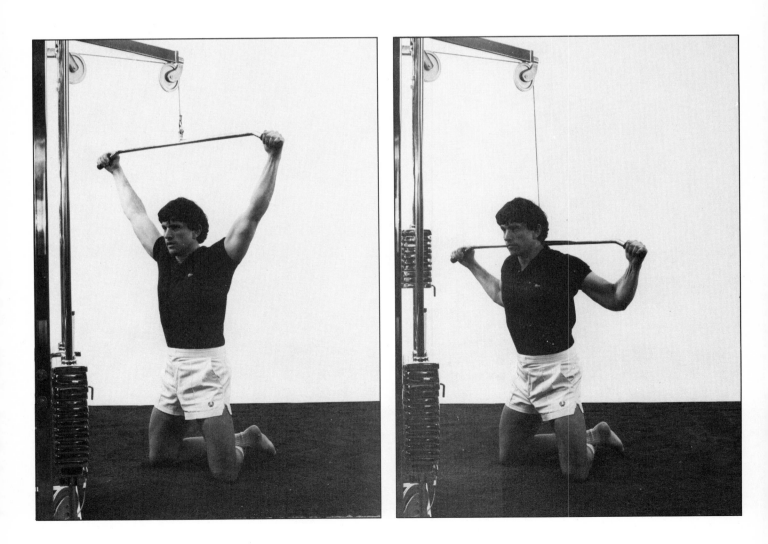

Back

Shoulders

111. Standing Front Presses:
One set.
Ten repetitions.

Presses tone the deltoid muscles of the shoulders. This one is primarily for the front of the shoulders, while the next exercise is more for the middle and rear heads of the deltoids.

Stand at the pressing bar facing the machine, so that the bar is on a line with the front edges of your shoulders, with your feet spread shoulder width apart. Now press straight upward to a nearly full extension of your arms and let the weight smoothly back down for one rep. Don't arch your back or jerk at the weight going up, and don't just drop it on the way down. Keep the tension of the exercise in the front of your shoulders throughout each repetition.

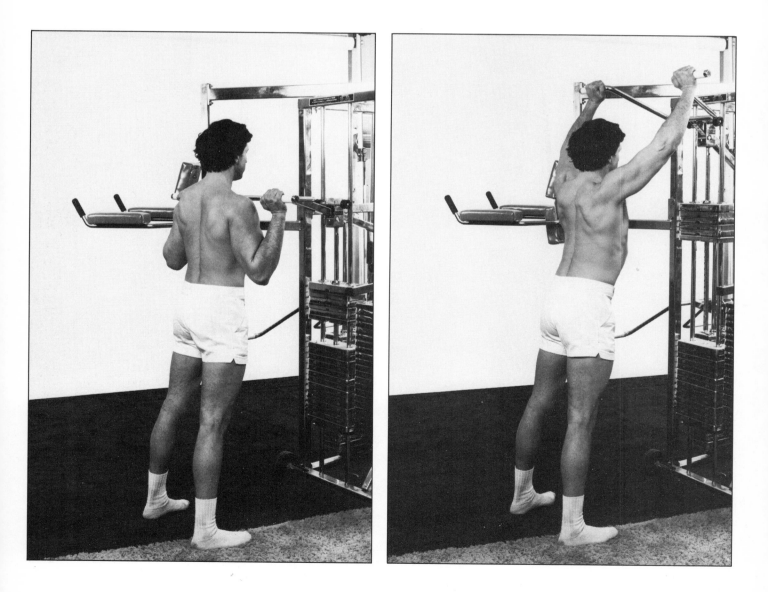

Shoulders

112. Behind-the-Neck Presses:
One set.
Fifteen repetitions.

For this rear-deltoid exercise, stand facing away from the machine with the bar at the rear of your shoulders. Press upward as in the previous exercise, and let the weight down slowly. Be sure to keep your back straight.

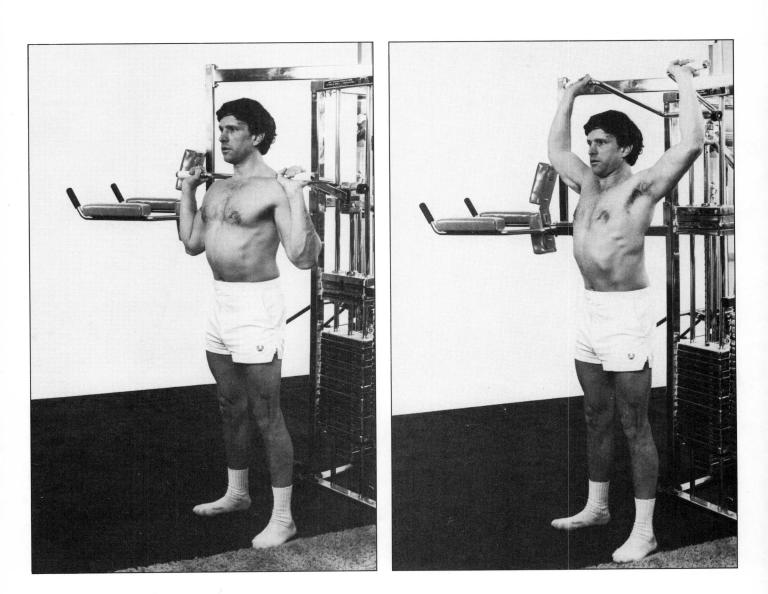

Arms

113. Curls:
One set.
Ten repetitions.

Next to the dorsi-bar position is a cable-and-pulley system at the bottom of the machine that can be used with either a bar attached to a length of chain or two handle grips. For this exercise, which tones the biceps at the front of the upper arms, you will want to use the bar.

Stand with your feet less than shoulder width apart and a foot to eighteen inches back from the base of the machine. Hold the bar with your hands about midway on either grip and your arms slightly bent at the elbows. Keep your back straight and don't move your upper body as you curl the bar up to touch your chest and lower it again slowly, for one repetition. Your elbows should remain still and close to your sides both going up and coming down.

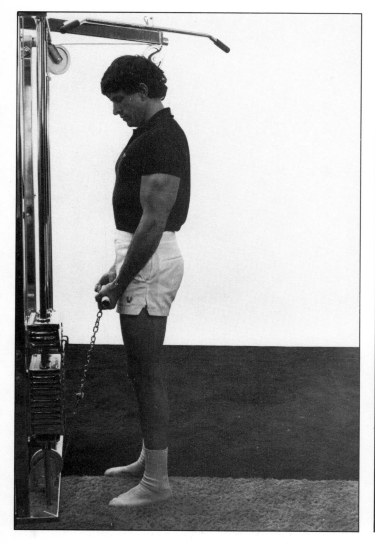
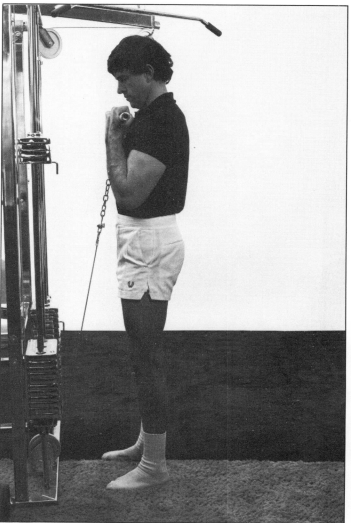

Arms

114. Triceps Presses:
One set.
Twenty repetitions.

For this exercise, which tones the backs of the arms, go back to the high-bar-and-cable station. Stand with your feet shoulder width apart and take a narrow grip on the bar. Keeping your back and upper arms straight, and your elbows close to your side and still, push the bar down toward the floor to just above waist height—this will be the top position for each repetition. Now continue to push the bar down, feeling the strain at the rear of your upper arms, until your elbows are almost but not quite locked. Then slowly let it up again to just above your waist for one repetition. *Think* the work into the triceps.

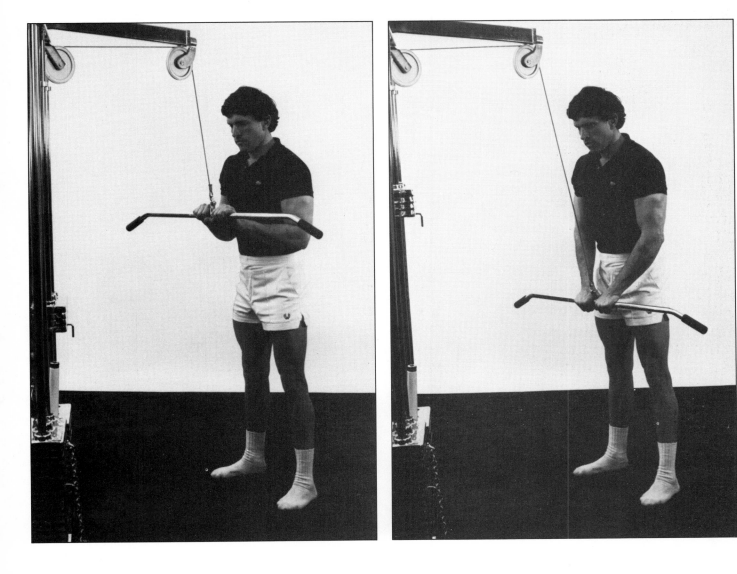

Program Eight
(Intermediate)
Target Time:
Twenty-two minutes

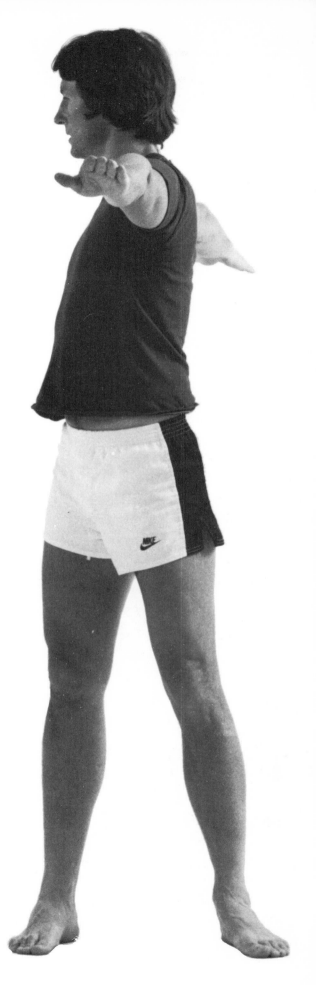

Waist

115. Bent-Leg Sit-ups:
One set.
Fifty repetitions.

This sit-up is particularly good for toning the waist, because it keeps tension on the muscles all the way through each repetition, and tension is what tones.

Put the slantboard into the first or lowest hole on its connecting post and sit on it with your feet under the rollers, your knees bent, and your arms at your sides. Keeping your hands by your hips, go back until your lower back touches the board, then sit back up and tense your stomach muscles at the top of the rep. The more tension you put on your waist through the set, the better.

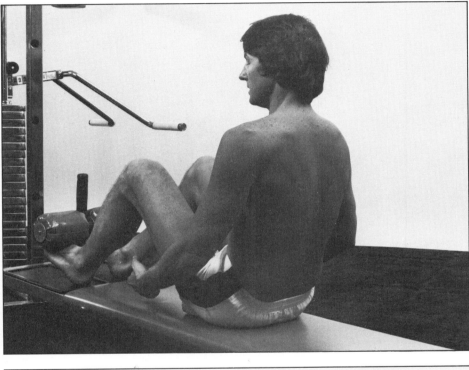

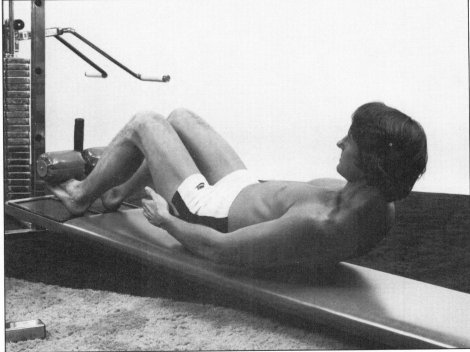

Waist

116. Knee-ins:
One set.
Twenty-five repetitions.

This is a terrific exercise for the lower abdominals, as well as for working out a stiff lower back.

Put the slantboard flat on the ground and lie on it with your hands under your buttocks. Raise your legs six to twelve inches off the board, and don't let them down again until the end of the set. Keep your legs together and bring your knees in toward your chest as far as you can, then straighten your legs slowly, for one repetition.

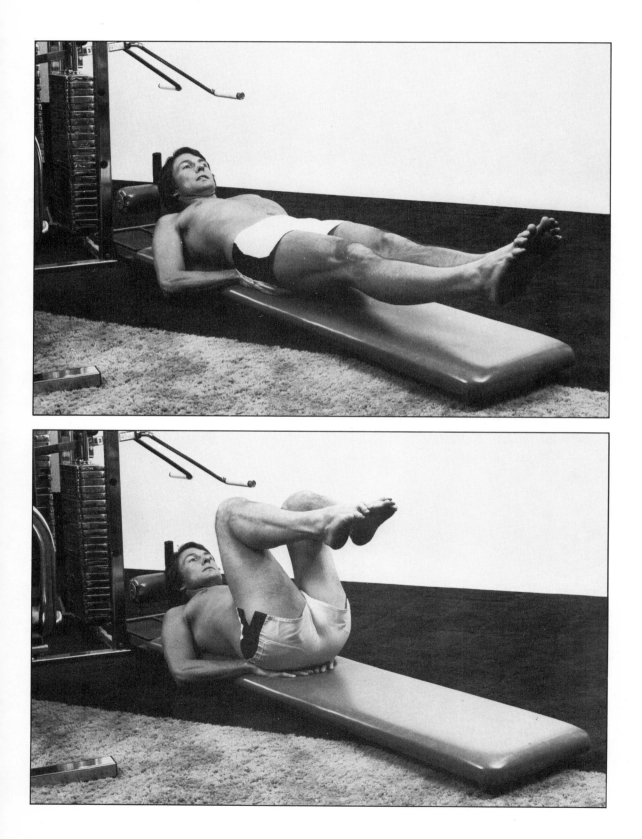

Waist

117. Side Bends and Twists:
One set.
Fifteen repetitions.

This four-part exercise is for hardening the intercostal and oblique muscles at the sides of the waist. It's a good exercise for overall flexibility and loosening the lower back.

Stand with your feet shoulder width apart, your arms held out horizontally at your sides. Movement one: Bend at the waist as far as you can to the right, keeping your arms in line, then come back up to vertical. Movement two: Do the same thing to the other side. Movement three: Arms in line, twist as far as you can to the right, letting your whole upper body come around. Movement four: Twist all the way around to the left; then go back to the original position, for one repetition. Keep your legs straight throughout.

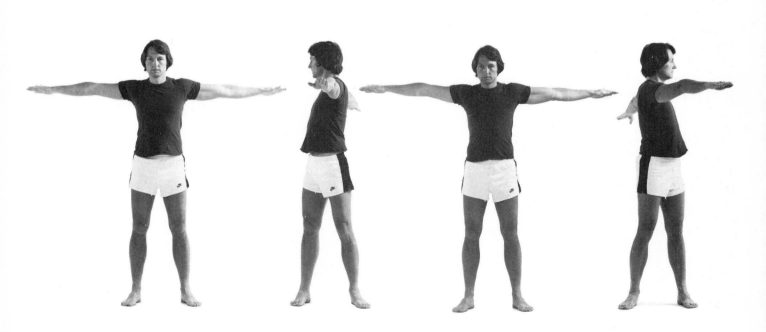

Legs and Buttocks

118. Leg Extensions:
One set.
Twenty repetitions.

This is an excellent exercise for hardening the frontal thighs, and for all sports. A month or so before ski season I start doing three sets of these a day, and though I may not ski any better because of them I know that my legs will take anything I put them to.

Sit on the leg machine shown here with your back straight and holding the bench. Lift your legs just enough to engage the weight, and don't let the weight all the way back down again until the last repetition. Keep your upper legs and torso still and bring your lower legs up to full extension, then lower slowly, for one repetition.

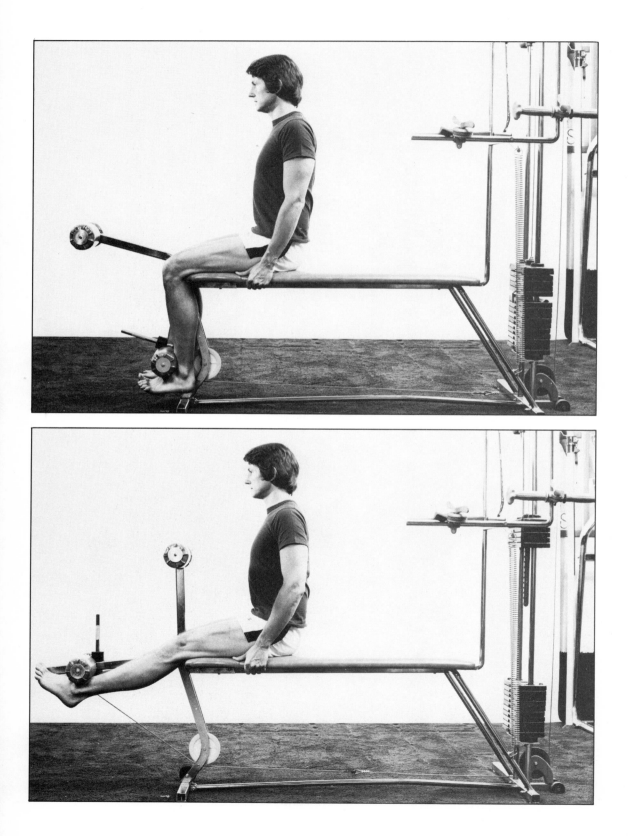

Legs and Buttocks

119. Leg Curls:
One set.
Twenty repetitions.

This tones the biceps femoris at the back of the thighs and the buttocks.

Lie on your stomach on the leg machine with your head and chest raised and your heels hooked under the top bars of the machine. Curl your heels up toward your buttocks, coming to or just past the vertical with your lower legs. Lower your legs again slowly, and don't quite let the weights touch the stationary plates before beginning your second rep. Be sure to keep your hips flat on the bench throughout.

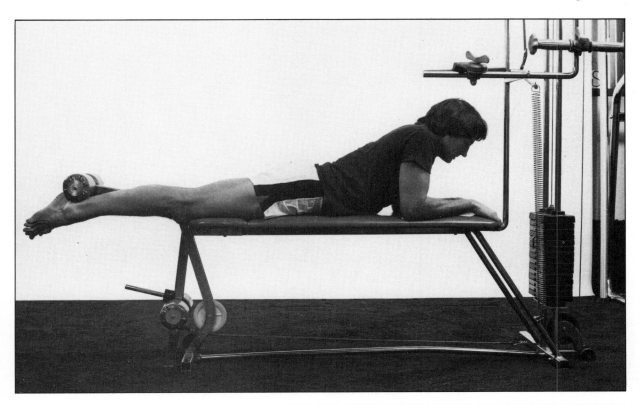

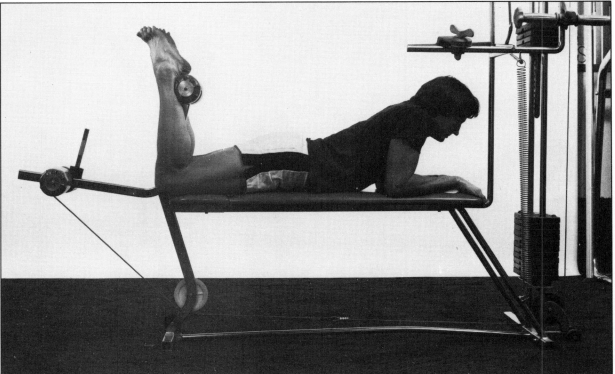

Legs and Buttocks

120. Hip Sweeps:
One set.
Ten repetitions to each side.

This is very good for toning the lower back and the sides of the waist and, particularly, the hips. It is also excellent for your flexibility.

Stand as shown with your hands clasped over your head and your left leg fully extended to the side, foot resting on the hyperextension pad. Sweep to the left and touch your left toe, then down to touch the floor in front of your right toe. Come vertical again for one repetition to that side. Do ten, then go to the other side of the hyperextension rack and do ten with the right leg extended.

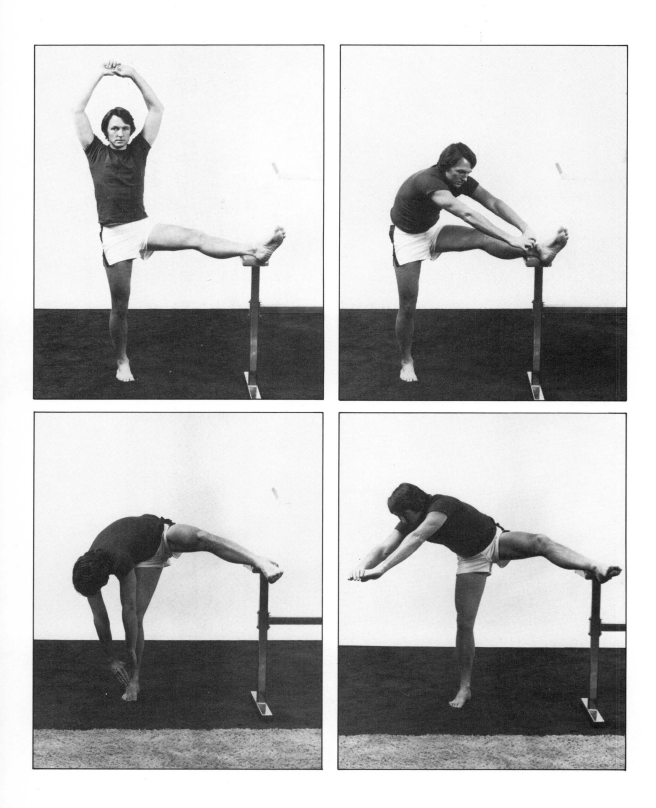

Legs and Buttocks

121. Calf Raises:
One set.
Twenty repetitions.

For this calf-toning and -shaping exercise, sit at the leg-press station with the seat in the second position back. Keep your back straight and press out with your legs to an almost full extension. Now slide your feet down the metal rests until only the balls of your feet remain on them. This is your first position. Then push with your toes, as if you were trying to point your feet, to the full stretch of your calf muscles. Hold it there for a count of two before coming back to the first position, for one repetition.

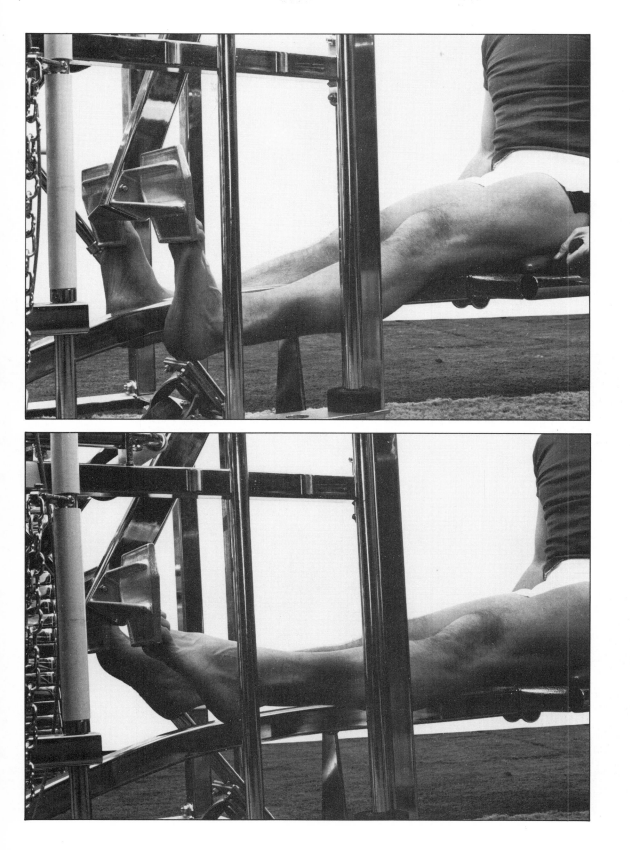

Legs and Buttocks

Chest

122. Bench Presses:
One set.
Twenty repetitions.

This press is almost identical to the one shown in the previous program (see Exercise 107). You do it holding the bars toward the outsides of the grips. Your hands are about level with your shoulders. Here you concentrate more toning stress on the pectoral muscle by putting your feet up on the bench.

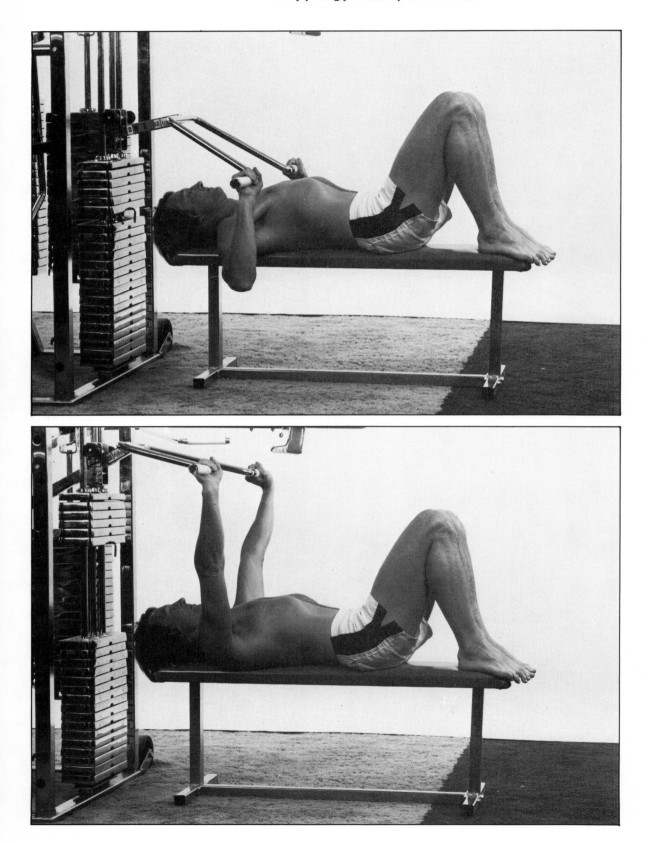

Chest

123. Lying Cable Flies:
One set.
Fifteen repetitions.

Though this exercise takes a bit of fooling around with the machine to organize, it is a wonderful chest-hardener.

Put a bench between the main machine and the leg machine and attach a metal handle to each of the two lower cable-pulley systems. Raise the handles until the weight is just engaged and use this as the first position for each rep. Keeping your arms bent slightly, bring your hands almost together in an arc, then lower your arms again slowly for one repetition. You should feel the exercise in the outside wings of your pectorals.

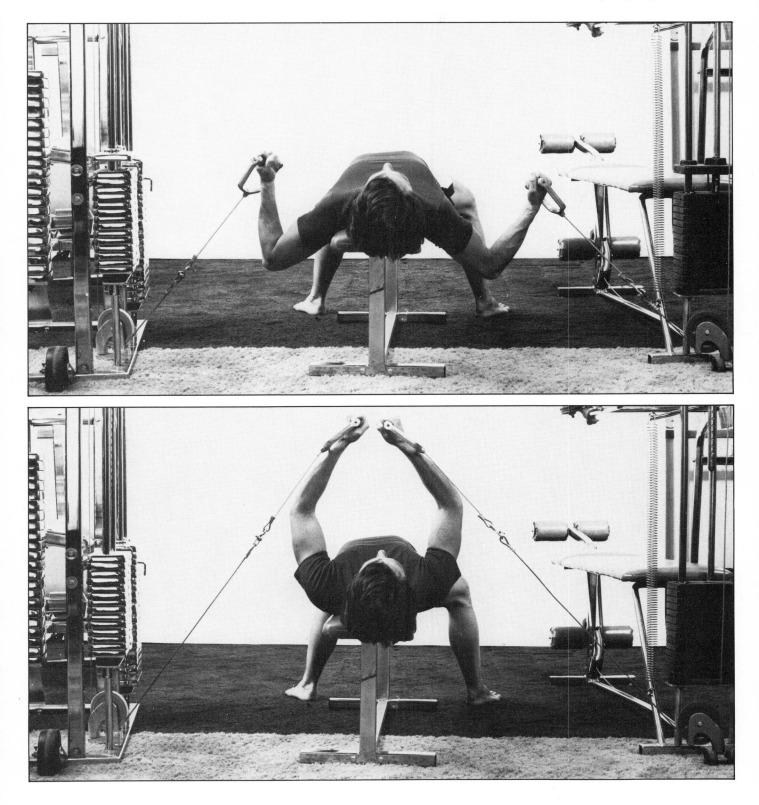

Back

124. Front Lat Pull-downs:
One set.
Twenty repetitions.

This exercise is for toning the upper back, particularly the latissimus dorsi muscles. Do it as described and shown for Exercise 110, except that here you should sit rather than kneel beneath the bar and pull it down in *front* of your head to touch your upper chest.

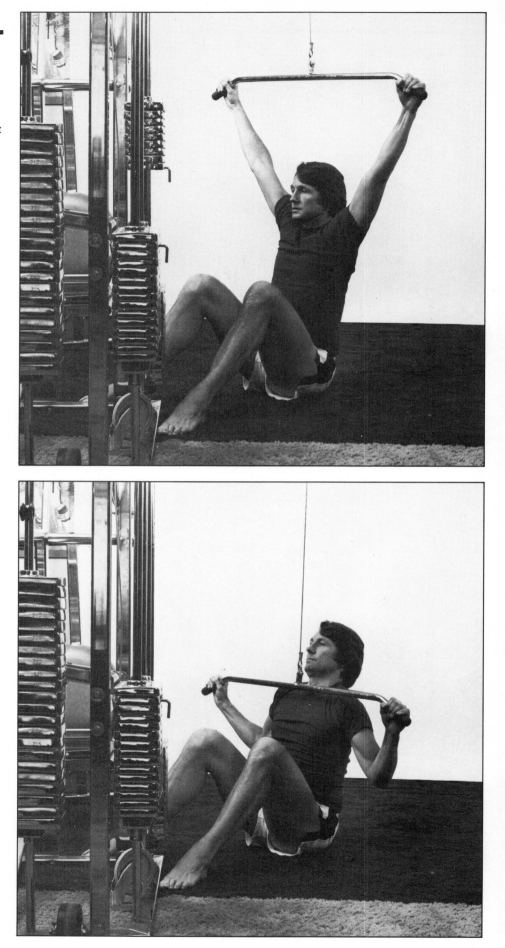

Back

125. Seated Pull-tos:
One set.
Twenty repetitions.

For the upper and lower back. Sit at the cable-pulley station shown here, your feet separated from the base of the machine by a block of wood, preferably in a T shape. Keep your back straight, and your arms extended, and pull the bar back just enough to engage the weight. This is your first position. Now pull the bar in to your stomach, letting your back do the work, and let it smoothly back out for one rep. Keep your upper body still throughout and concentrate the exercise into your back.

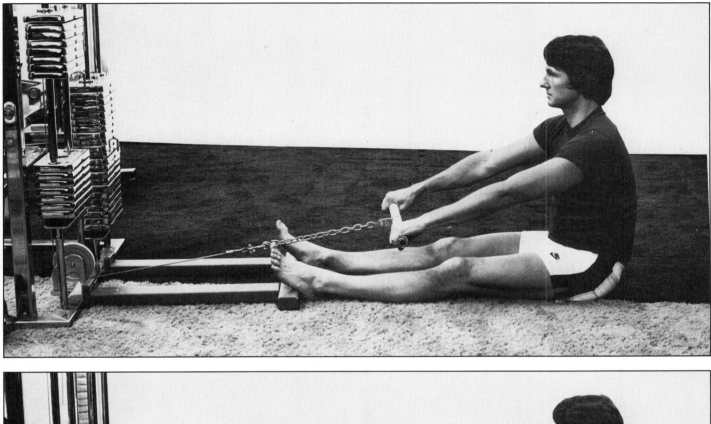

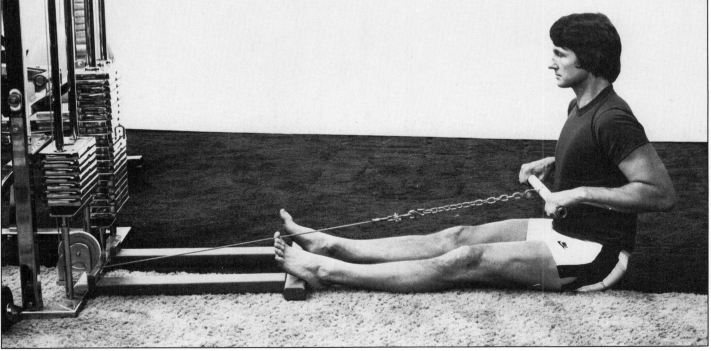

Shoulders

126. Seated Presses:
One set.
Twenty repetitions.

This exercise tones all three heads of the deltoid muscles of the shoulders.

Sit at the shoulder-press station facing the machine with the bar at the front edge of your shoulders. Keep your back straight. Press straight up for ten repetitions. Now turn around on the stool and face away from the machine; the bar now should lie along the rear line of your shoulders. Do ten more repetitions in this position, again holding your back absolutely straight.

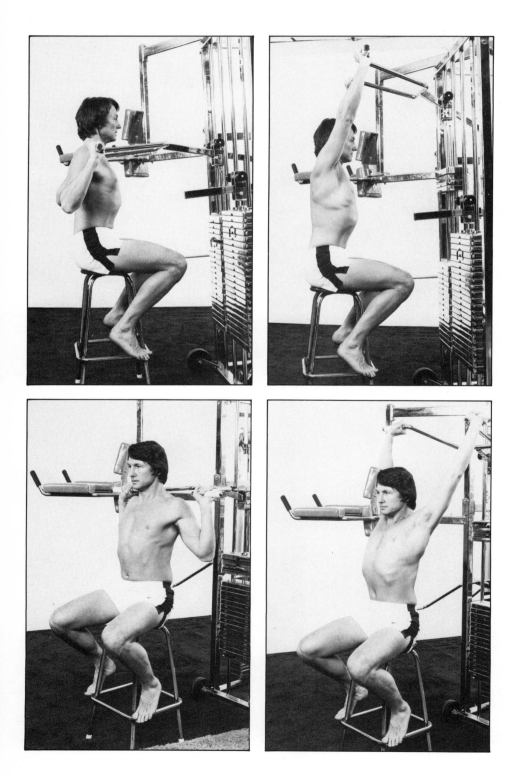

Shoulders

127. Side Laterals:
One set.
Ten repetitions to each side.

This is a good exercise for most sports and a fine overall shoulder toner. You will probably want to use a small amount of weight.

Stand with your feet spaced wider than your shoulders, your right side turned to the machine and your right foot about twelve inches from its base. Bend at the waist and take hold of the metal handle with your left hand. Pull it out and up, with your arm going straight out from your body and slightly bent at the elbow. Go up to where your upper arm is level with your back, then down again, smoothly, for one repetition.

If you can't pull the handle up this far, stand straight instead of bending at the waist and just pull it out a few inches at a time.

Do ten with your left arm, then turn around and do ten with your right.

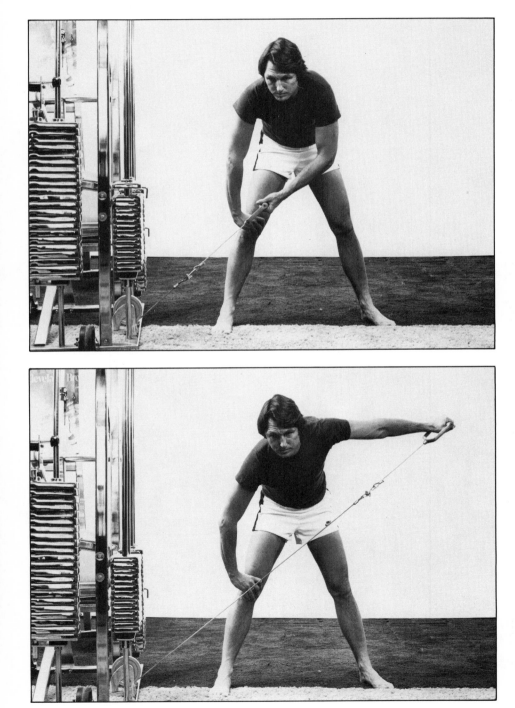

Arms

128. Curls:
One set.
Twenty repetitions.

For this biceps toner, sit on the stool in front of the low cable-pulley station, this time attached to the bar rather than to the handle grip.

Sit with your back straight, your knees only a few inches from the machine, holding the bar between your legs with your arms fully extended. Now curl the bar up to your chin, keeping your upper arms and back motionless, then lower it again slowly to a point just before the weights touch for one repetition. Do this exercise slowly and with good concentration.

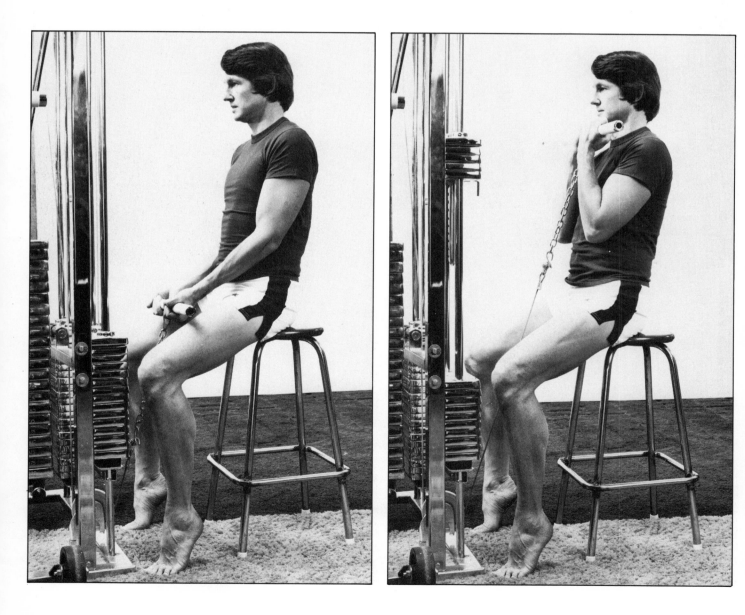

Arms

129. Triceps Presses:
One set.
Twenty repetitions.

For this exercise, which tones the backs of the arms, do the first ten repetitions exactly as described and shown for Exercise 114. Then without a break, bend over at the waist and hold the bar at the top of your head. Push your forearms straight down from there, hinging at the elbows and keeping your upper arms and body absolutely still. Let the bar slowly back to the top of your head for one repetition. Do ten of these too, for a set total of twenty reps.

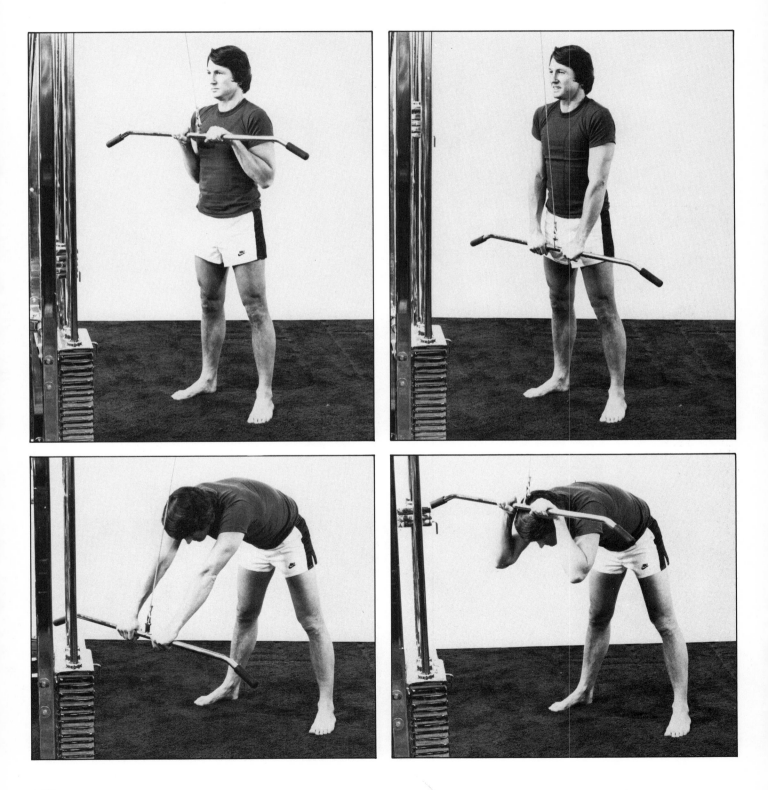

Program Nine

(Advanced)
Target Time:
Thirty-five minutes

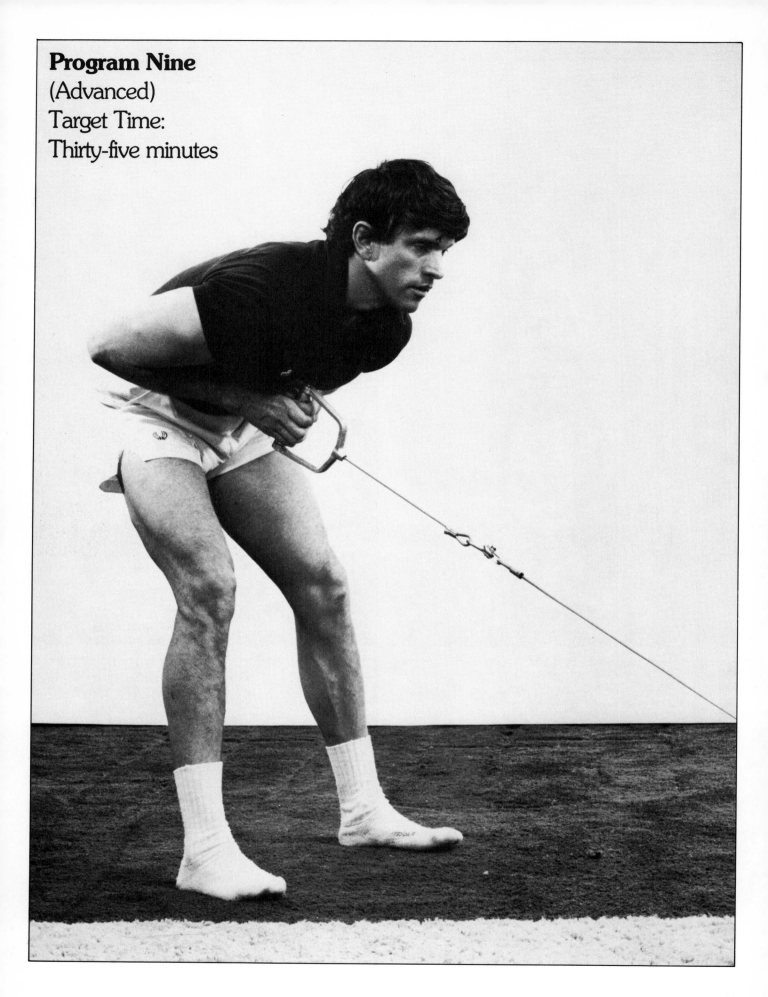

Waist

130. Bent-Leg Sit-ups:
One set.
One hundred repetitions.

Like all the exercises in this section, this is a more difficult form of a common movement, the purpose of this one being to tone the upper abdominals.

Put the slantboard into the first or lowest hole on the post and sit on it with your knees bent, your hands locked behind your head. Go down until you touch your lower back, then sit smoothly back up for one repetition. Do these quickly and keep tension on the stomach muscles throughout, particularly at the top of the repetition.

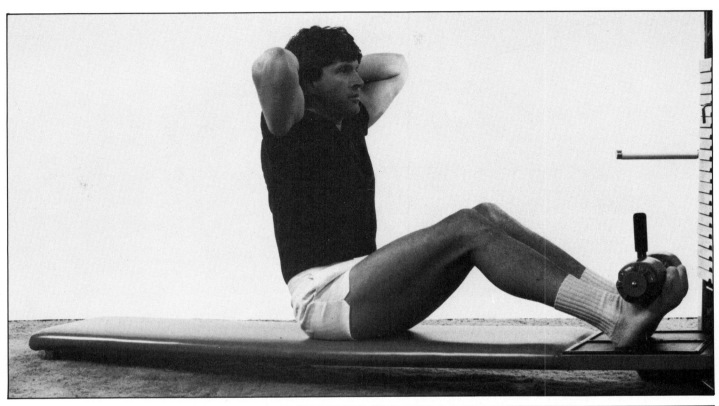

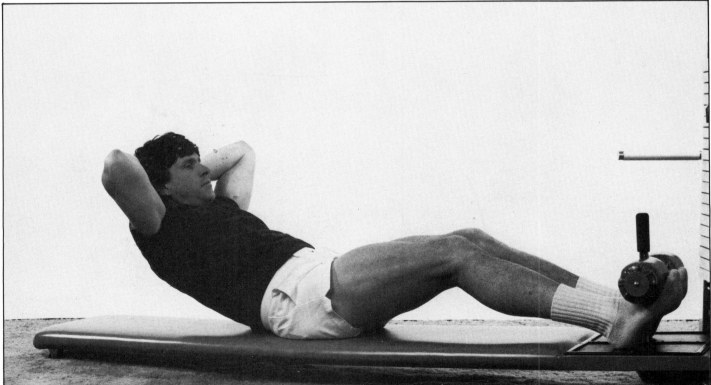

Waist

131. Hanging Leg-ins:
One set.
Twenty-five repetitions.

This exercise is wonderful for hardening the lower abdominals and for spinal flexibility. When my lower back is particularly stiff, this is what I use to loosen it.

Hang from the station shown here with your knees bent. Using your stomach muscles, draw your knees up toward your chest as far as they will go, then smoothly lower your legs to the first position, keeping your upper body quiet and tension on the muscles throughout.

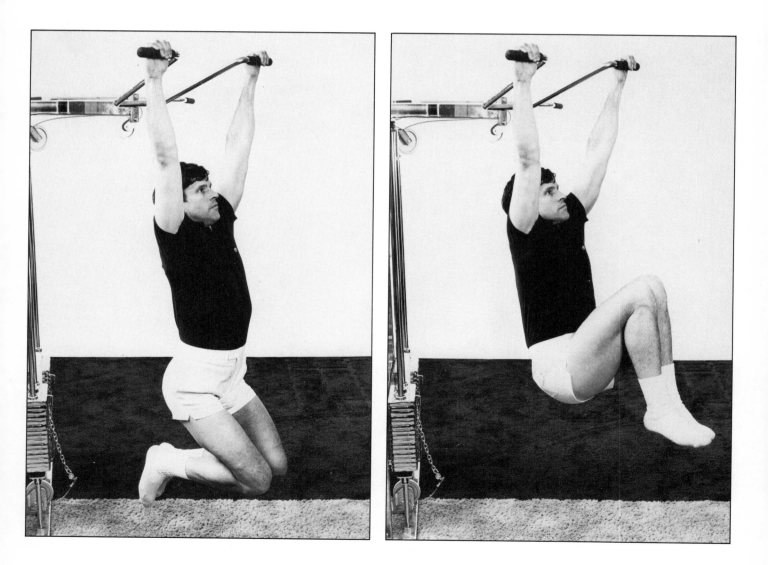

Waist

132. Side Bends with Cable:
One set.
Twenty repetitions to each side.

This exercise works the oblique and intercostal muscles along the sides of the waist. To do it, stand at the lower cable station with your right side to the machine, your feet shoulder width apart and eighteen inches away from the base. Holding the handle grip, engage the weight and bend to your left, letting your left hand drop below your knee, and stretching the muscles along your right side. Go back up smoothly, for one rep. Do twenty to each side.

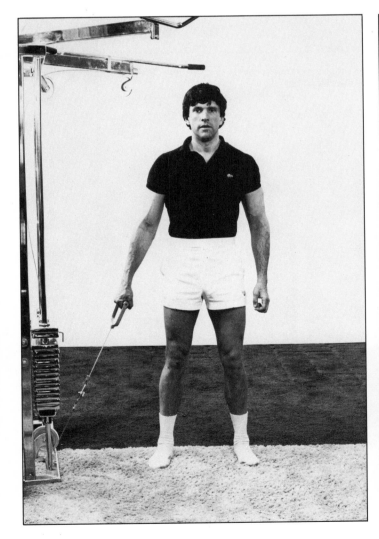 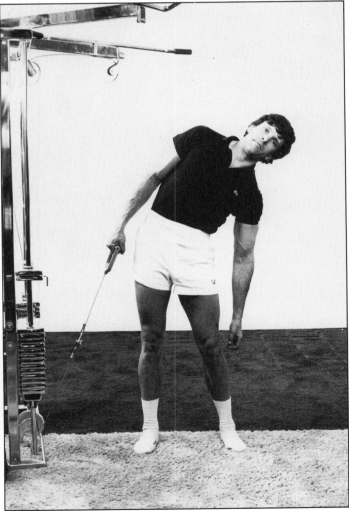

Waist

133. Back Bends with Cable:
One set.
Twenty repetitions.

This is a good flexibility and lower-back exercise and is good for all sports, particularly tennis. It is also a fine stomach hardener, toning the whole frontal length of the waist.

Stand as shown here, feet twelve inches apart and six or so from the base of the machine, holding the bar connected to the lower cable station with your palms facing downward. There should be a slight bend in your elbows, and they should be touching your sides. Engage the weight and bend back as far as you can at the waist, leaving your arms in their original position. Then come smoothly back to vertical for one repetition.

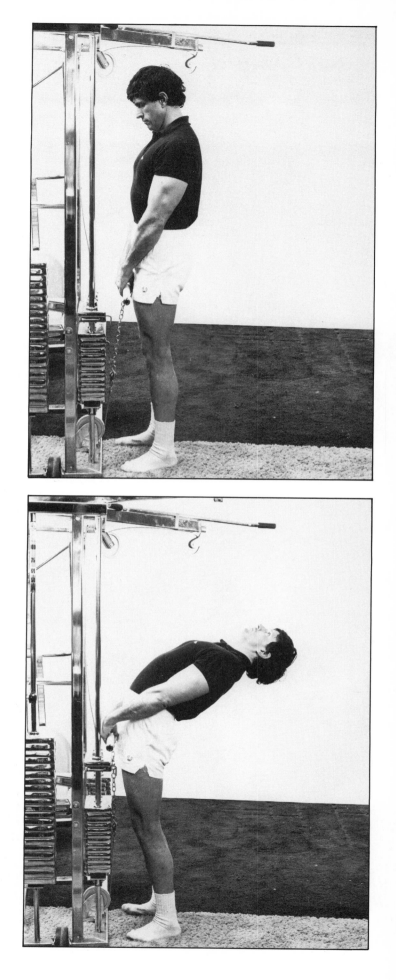

134. Alternating Leg Presses:

One set.
Twenty repetitions with each leg.

This is a fine toner of the upper legs and hips. To do it, sit at the leg-press station with the seat in the closest position to the machine. Keep your back straight. Alternate pressing the weight with your right and left legs, not quite locking the knee on each extension and not quite letting the weight touch the other plates on the retraction. Keep your buttocks on the seat. Do twenty with each leg.

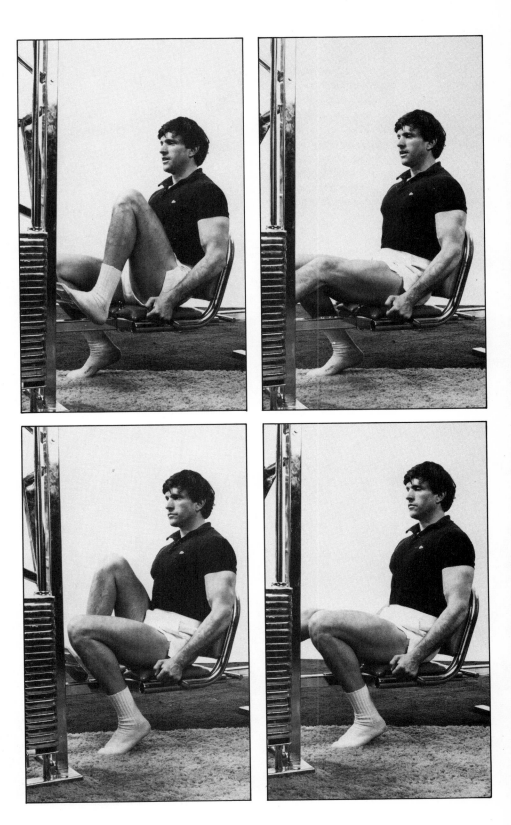

Legs and Buttocks

135. Alternating Leg Extensions:
One set.
Twenty repetitions with each leg.

By using the block here you put more stress on the lower quadriceps muscles of the thigh, and by alternating one leg at a time you locate the exercise more specifically in that area. This exercise is an ace for all sports.

Sit on the bench with a two-by-four block under your legs just behind the knees and both feet under the bottom bars. Lift the bars just enough to engage the weight, and use that as your original position. Now bring up the weight with your right leg (your left leg following) to an almost full extension, then lower; then raise the weight with your left leg and lower for one repetition with each leg. Do twenty with each, alternating the reps.

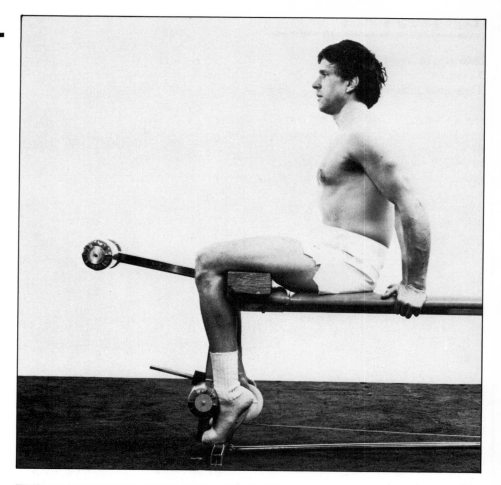

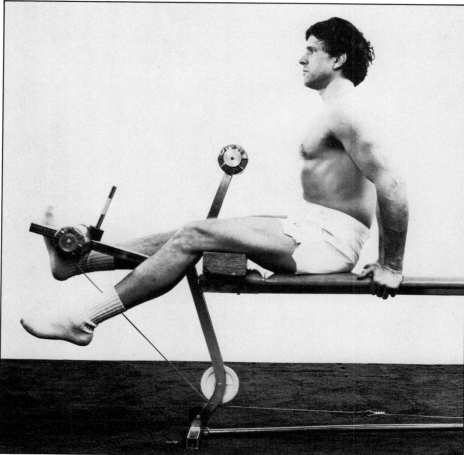

Legs and Buttocks

136. Alternating Leg Curls:
One set.
Fifteen repetitions with each leg.

You do this exercise, for toning the backs of the thighs, in the same way as described for Exercise 119, by bringing the weight up smoothly toward your buttocks, except that here you curl the weight with one leg at a time (the other following up), alternating for fifteen repetitions with each. Remember to keep your hips flat on the bench, and to think the exercise into your hamstrings.

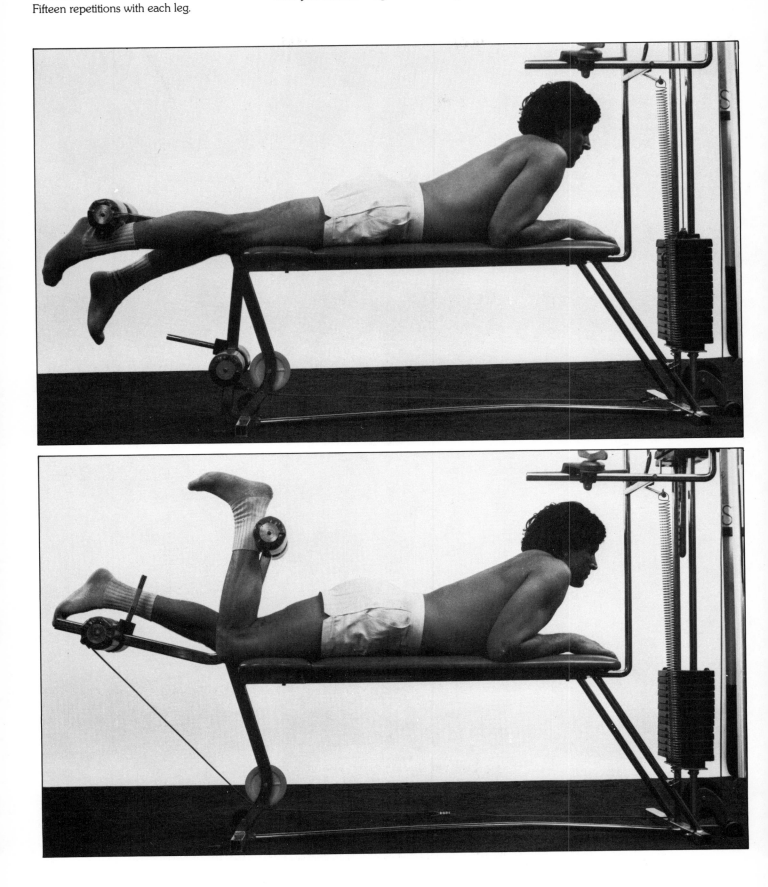

137. One-Leg Calf Raises:
One set.
Thirty repetitions with each leg.

These calf raises—for shaping and toning the lower legs—are done using the shoulder-press station as shown for Exercise 106.

Stand as shown with the ball of your right foot and an inch or two of your instep on a block. Drop your heel so that it is touching, or just off, the floor. Now stand up smoothly onto your toes and hold the movement at full extension for a couple of seconds before dropping back down for one repetition. Do thirty reps with each calf, and use as much weight as you can.

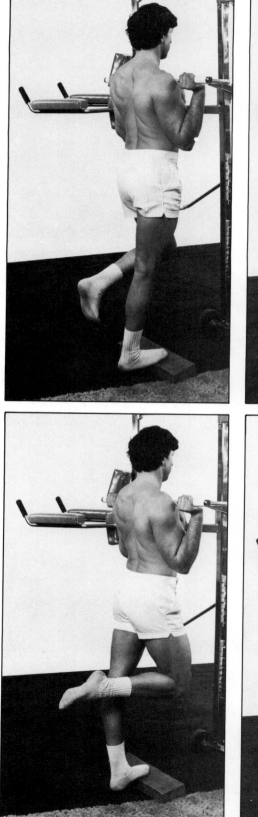
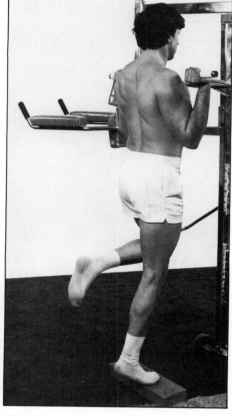
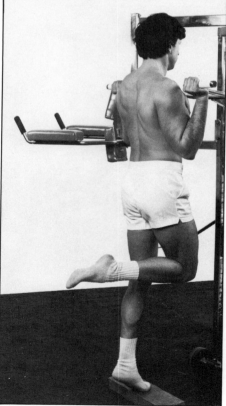

Chest

138. Inclined Bench Presses:
One set.
Twenty-five repetitions.

This is a particularly effective variation of the bench press because it isolates well on the pectoral muscle and really stretches it out at the bottom of each repetition.

Put the head of the bench on a block of wood or something four to six inches high and situate it close to the weight plates. Lie on the bench with your head close to the weights so that the bars are in line with your lower chest. When you grip the bars your hands should be lower than your chest. Lift the bars just enough to engage the weight and use that as your bottom position for each rep. Now push straight up to almost a full extension, and lower to the first position for one repetition. Really let your pectorals stretch on this one.

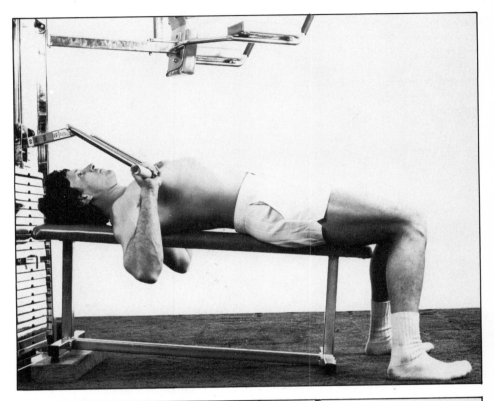

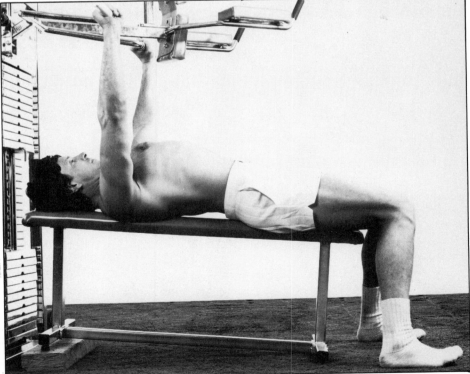

Chest

139. Dips:
One set.
Fifteen repetitions.

Dips are a terrific chest-hardening exercise but they are difficult to do strictly if your chest is not in very good shape, so both a strict and a not-so-strict method of doing them are offered here. For the strict method, go up on the dipping bars with arms extended, feet crossed, and gripping the bars with the thumbs forward. Now, bending your lower legs and rocking your upper body a little forward, dip down until your chest is even or below the bars and push smoothly back up.

For the easier alternative method, stand on a bench or stool and help yourself rise with your legs, but using them as little as possible. However you do it, make the chest, not the shoulders and triceps, do the work; concentrate the exercise there.

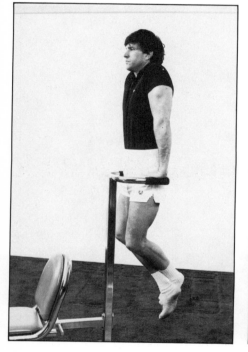
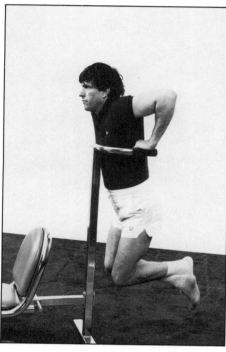
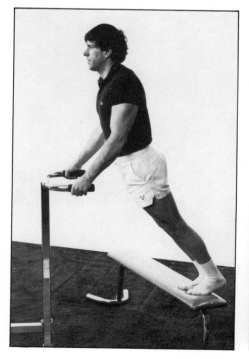
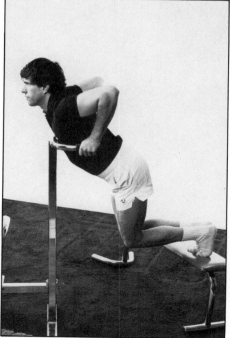

Back

140. Hyperextensions:
One set.
Fifteen repetitions.

Hyperextensions tone the lower-back muscles and the buttocks. They are also very good for lower-back problems and for your flexibility.

Position yourself on the hyperextension rack as shown, with your head and back lowered toward the floor, your hands clasped at the small of your back. Now stretch upward as high as you can, keeping your head high, and lower yourself slowly to the first position, for one repetition. Do these slowly.

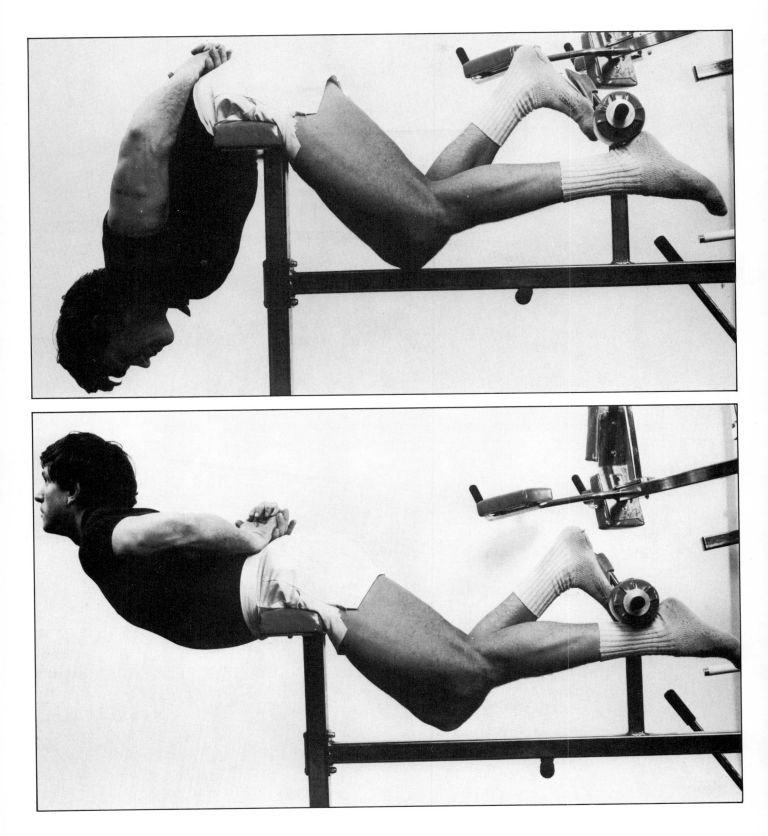

Back

141. Cable Pulls:
One set.
Repetitions as given below.

This is another exercise whose strict form may be too difficult for some people, so an easier variation is also offered. Both exercises work on the latissimus dorsi and other muscles of the upper back.

For the strict form, stand bent at the waist in front of the low cable station as shown. Start with your right arm lying on your right knee and your left arm extended, hand holding the handle grip. Engage the weight and pull back, putting the work along the left side of your back, until the grip touches your chest. Do fifteen reps with your left arm, then reverse your position and do fifteen with your right.

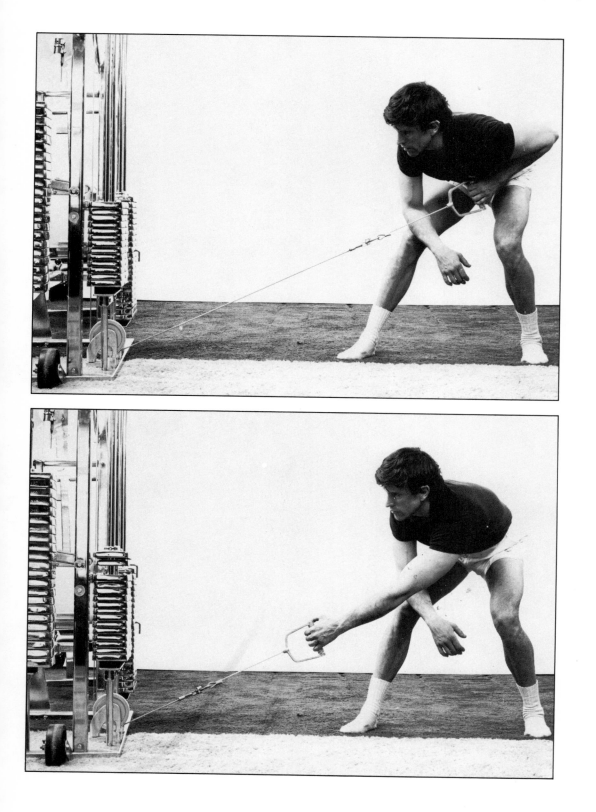

For the easier version, stand as shown
with both hands holding a single handle grip.
Pull it straight into your chest—again putting
the strain on the sides of the back—and let it
back out slowly for one rep. Do twenty-five
of these.

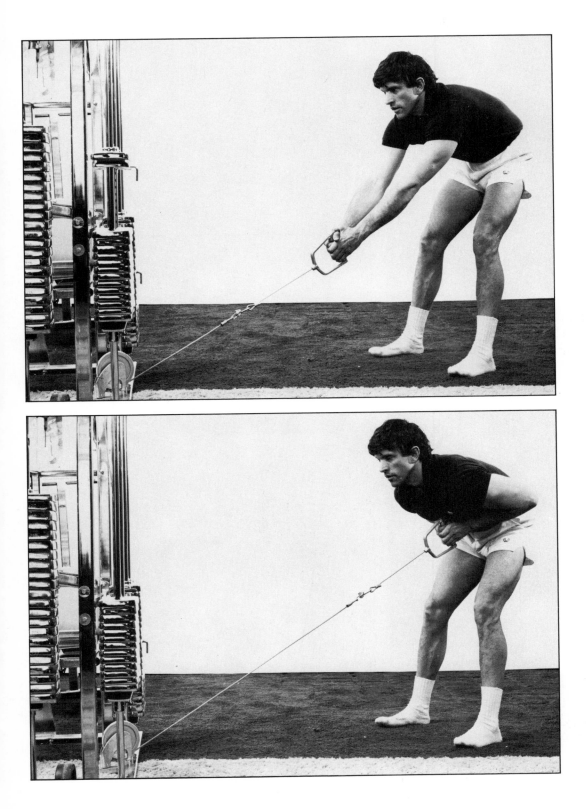

Shoulders

142. Seated Presses:
One set.
Forty repetitions.

Do this front and rear deltoid-toning exercise exactly as described for Exercise 126, except that here do twenty repetitions with the bars behind your neck and then, without stopping, twenty with them in front. Do them fast, and during each group of repetitions don't let your weight touch the unused plates beneath.

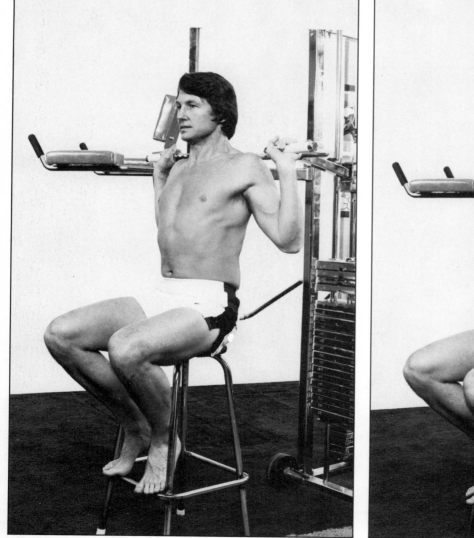
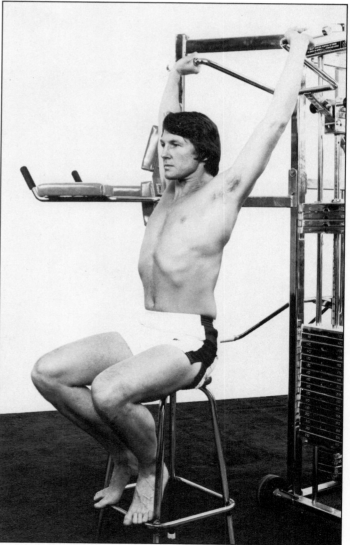

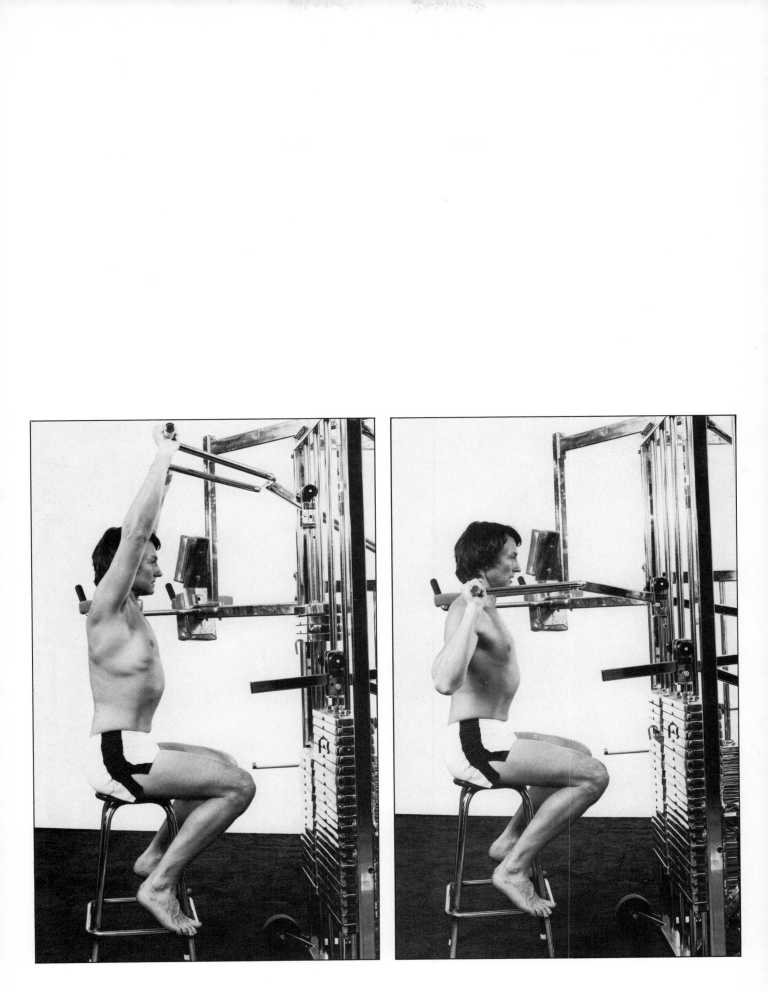

Shoulders

143. Front Flies with Cable:
One set.
Twenty repetitions.

This exercise tones the frontal deltoids and the trapezius muscles at the base of the neck.

Stand with your feet a foot to eighteen inches apart, gripping the bar attachment to the low cable station, your hands close together. Step back from the machine until you engage the weight and use that as your first position. Now, holding your back straight and your arms in a line, lift the bar up to eye level and lower again slowly for one repetition. Do these smoothly and with concentration.

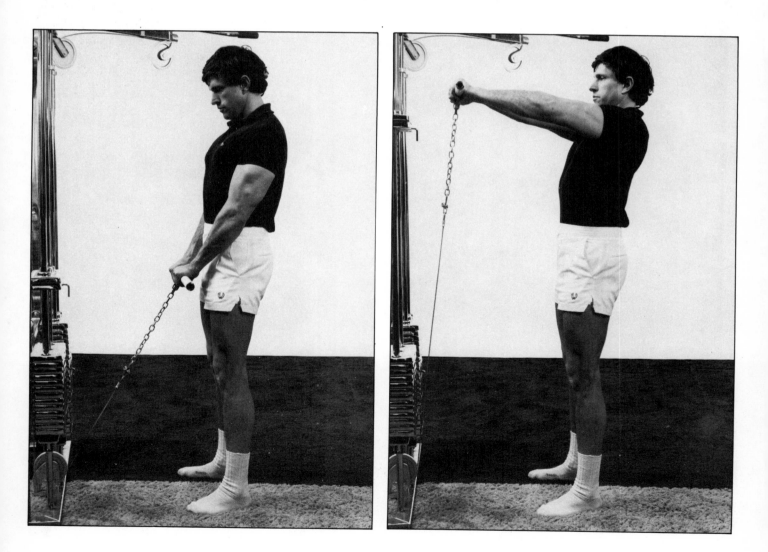

Arms

144. Lying Curls with Cable:
One set.
Twenty-five repetitions.

For this fine, strict biceps toner, lie on your back with your feet against the base of the machine in front of the low cable station. Hold the bar attachment with your arms fully extended, hands inside your hips and gripping the bar at either end. Keeping your upper arms absolutely still and your back flat on the floor, curl the bar up to the top of your chest and let it smoothly back down for one repetition. The weight should be engaged at the bottom position of each rep.

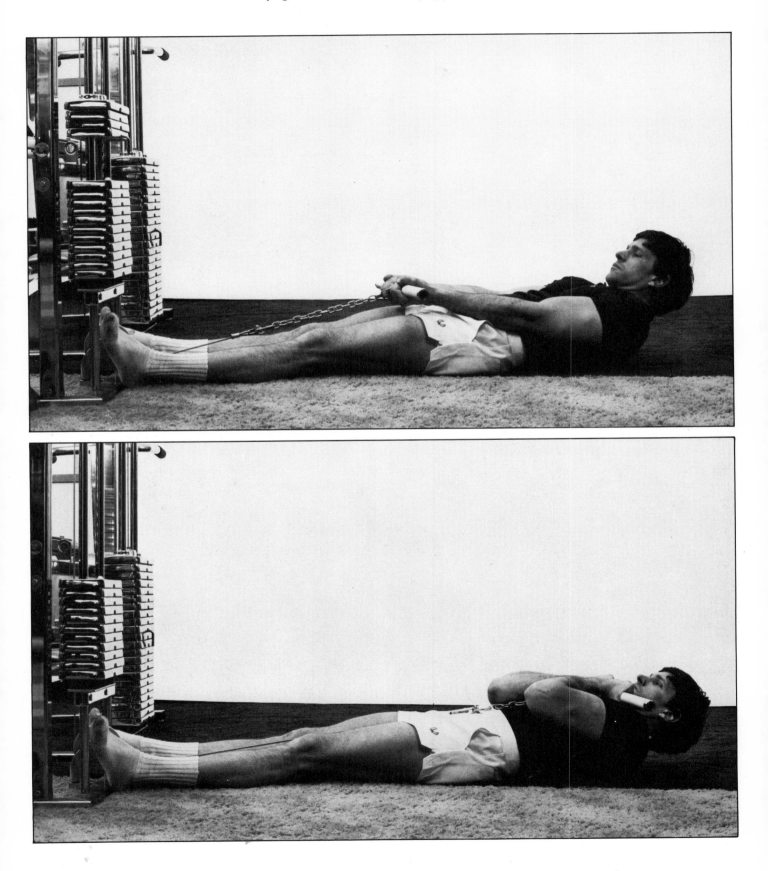

This tones and hardens the backs of the arms.

145. Seated Triceps Presses with Cable:
One set.
Twenty-five repetitions with each arm.

Sit close to the machine and facing away from it, the bench or stool at the low cable station. Hold one of the handle grips in your left hand just behind your left ear. Lift the handle until the weight is engaged. Now, keeping your elbow and upper arm still and your back straight, push your lower arm up to an almost full extension, then lower it again for one rep with that arm. Do twenty-five repetitions with each arm.

If you can't do this exercise as described with one arm, use both of them at the same time and do thirty repetitions.

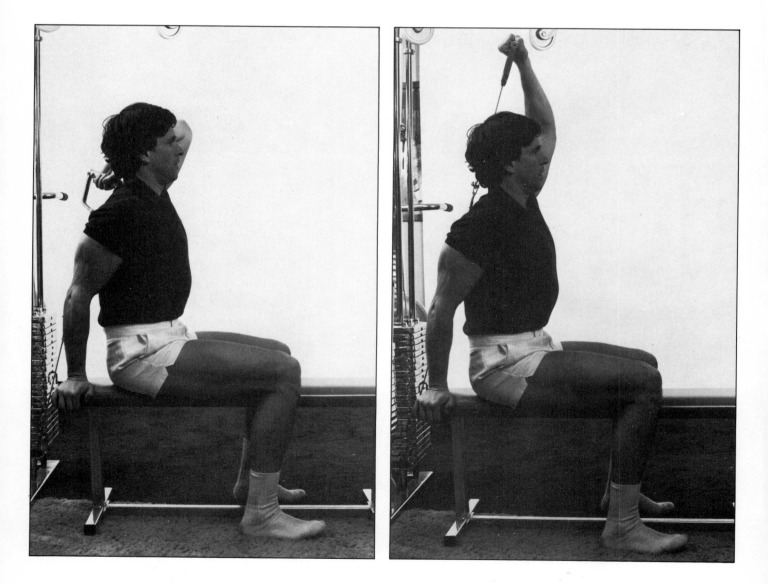

146. Reverse Dips:
One set.
Fifteen repetitions.

These dips are for toning the triceps as opposed to the pectorals, and they are done with the hands reversed (thumbs to the rear) as shown. Otherwise they are done exactly as are the dips in Exercise 139 of this program.

This is a difficult exercise if your triceps are anything less than mighty hard. If you can't do it the way it is shown here, modify the exercise with the same variation shown for Exercise 139, by keeping your legs elevated on a stool or a bench and letting them help you rise, but only slightly.

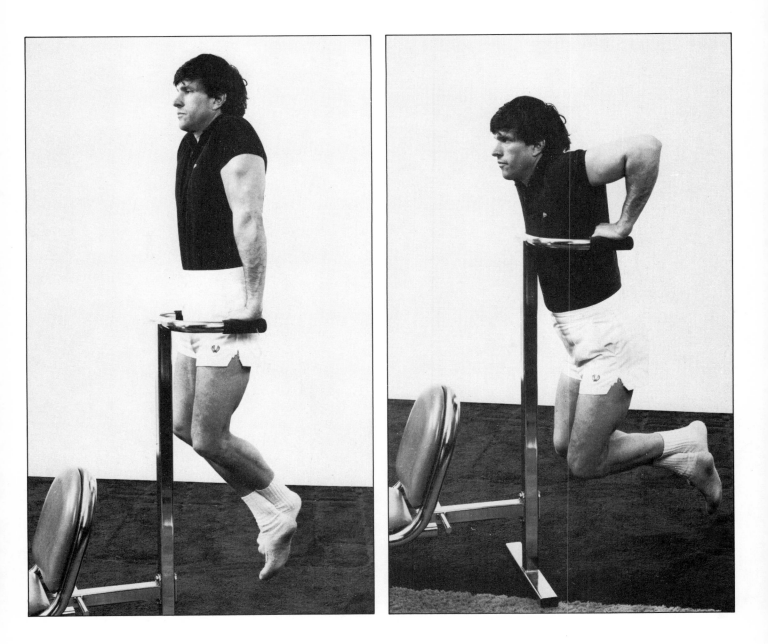

·IV·
MUSCLE CHART AND DIETARY TIPS

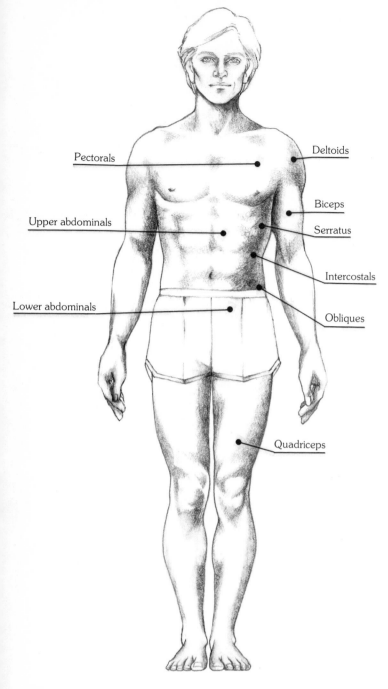

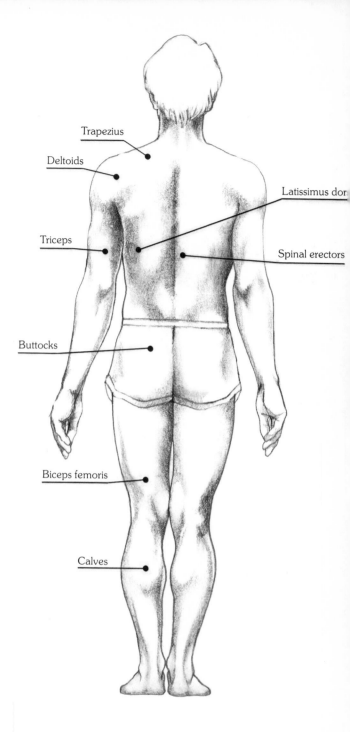

Muscle Chart

Muscle Group	Name of Muscle	Location in Body
I Waist	Lower abdominals	Between navel and pelvis
	Upper abdominals	Between sternum and navel
	Intercostals	Upper sides of waist
	Obliques	Lower sides of waist
II Legs & Buttocks	Buttocks	Sort of on top of the legs in the back
	Quadriceps	Front of thighs
	Biceps femoris	Backs of thighs (hamstrings)
	Calves	Backs of lower legs

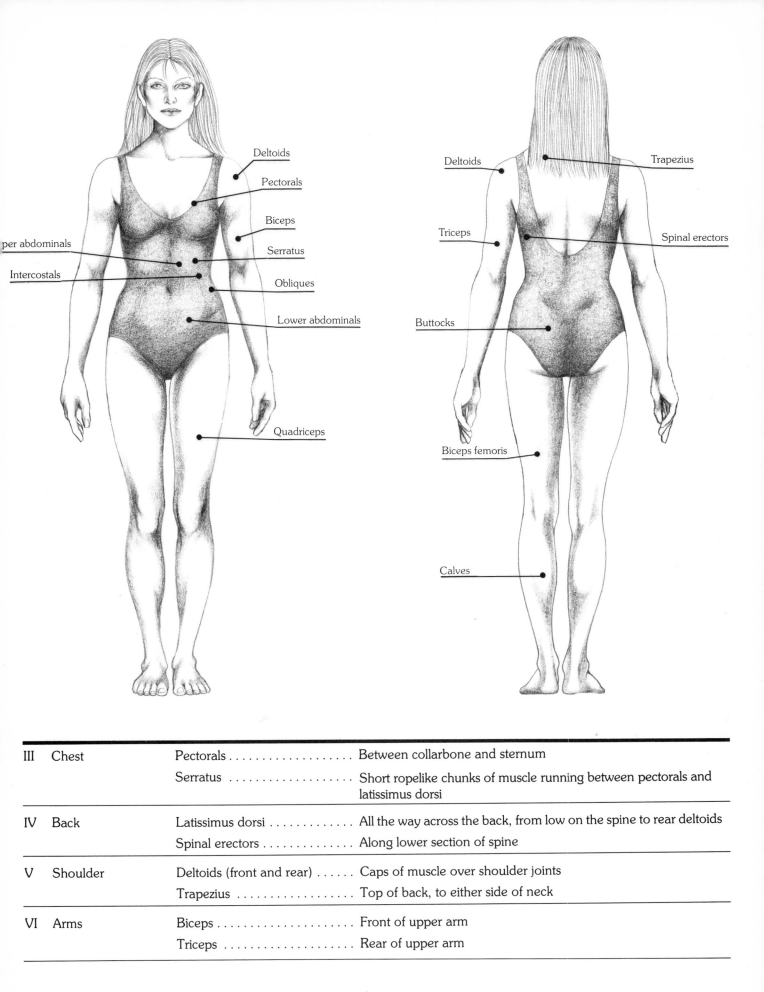

Deltoids

Pectorals

Biceps

Serratus

Obliques

Lower abdominals

per abdominals

Intercostals

Quadriceps

Deltoids

Trapezius

Triceps

Spinal erectors

Buttocks

Biceps femoris

Calves

III	Chest	Pectorals	Between collarbone and sternum
		Serratus	Short ropelike chunks of muscle running between pectorals and latissimus dorsi
IV	Back	Latissimus dorsi	All the way across the back, from low on the spine to rear deltoids
		Spinal erectors	Along lower section of spine
V	Shoulder	Deltoids (front and rear)	Caps of muscle over shoulder joints
		Trapezius	Top of back, to either side of neck
VI	Arms	Biceps	Front of upper arm
		Triceps	Rear of upper arm

Eating Hard

Personally, I dislike exercise books that go into a whole lot of cant about diet—the grams of animal proteins you should ingest every day, that sort of thing. I have the same objection to that approach to diet that I have to pornographic movies as an approach to sexual instruction: It's too schematic.

I believe in enjoying all kinds of food, and I love eating (and drinking) as much as anyone I know. But you can eat soft or eat hard, and if you want to stay hard, hard is the right way to eat.

It's not much of a sacrifice to eat hard—you can eat as much as you want that way, and though you do have to be a little selective you'll find after doing it for a while that the selection tends toward better-tasting and more satisfying foods. At least I find that. And this is a very personal list of tips, though some are less personal than others. None of them is a joke. Every one of them works for me (and many of them for other people I know), and I believe they will work for you too.

1. Contrary to what a lot of books will tell you, you *don't* have to eat an enormous breakfast every morning full of eggs and cream and dripping fats. That kind of breakfast usually gets you off on a soft, digestive slant to the day. Here is a good hard weekday breakfast: a glass of fresh-squeezed orange or grapefruit juice, for energy and a quick hop in your blood sugar level; half an English muffin spread with honey, for more energy, and roughage; and a cup of tea or coffee. Coffee, by the way, is harder than tea.

Beer for breakfast, like Hunter Thompson frequently has, is very soft, though he is not.

2. For breakfast and any other time, wheat germ is one of the hardest and best-tasting things there is. It is one of the few foods with vitamin E in it. It also has all the B vitamins except for B_{12}, and potassium, magnesium, zinc, and iron. It increases your stamina and fights stress and fatigue. Add it to your scrambled eggs when you make them on the week-

ends—also to ground chuck or round for meat loaf; to rice, wheat, and barley dishes; to bread. Eat a lot of it and get all that zinc and iron and everything working for you.

3. It should go without saying at this point in history that junk food is junk food. It is also extremely soft, so just don't eat it. Period. This includes all candy, except butterscotch balls, which are hard.

4. In addition to wheat germ, these are the other major hard foods: all kinds of meat except for pork (Canadian bacon is an exception); nuts, particularly cashews; cheese; all kinds of fish and shellfish; all kinds of poultry except for domestic turkeys; all vegetables; all fruits. Salads of almost any kind are particularly hard, and the hardest of all foods is wild game, which you should eat as often as you can, and with reverence.

5. Use fructose (fruit sugar) or honey—or anything else sweet—rather than refined white sugar. Don't use white flour either.

6. Desserts, unless they are of fruit, are by nature soft, but some are softer than others. Arnold Schwarzenegger thinks cake is better for you than pie, for instance. Indian pudding is fairly hard. Baked Alaska is hopelessly soft. For the most part, try to avoid desserts.

7. Try not to eat between meals. If you have to, eat fruit, nuts, or cheese. One of the hardest and best things you can eat between meals is Weaver's chicken loaf, but it is expensive and sometimes hard to find.

8. All proteins, animal and vegetable, are hard. Carbohydrates are more problematic. High-carbohydrate foods are good for energy and stamina, a hard characteristic; but too many or the wrong kind of carbs is definitely soft. A baked potato of average size has only eighty-five calories, and eaten with its skin on is very good carbs indeed. French fries are not. To my mind the three hardest high-carbohydrate foods of all are wild rice, avocados, and lima beans. For some reason most fats are hard, and if you are exercising regularly you don't have to worry about them. There has never been a harder people than the plains Indians of North

America, and they ate mostly fats. So do Eskimos, who are also very hard.

9. A certain amount of bread is OK, as long as it is whole wheat, rye, pumpernickel, or, best of all, glutenbread. Someone hard would rather slit his or her wrists than eat a piece of white bread.

10. A typical daily menu of hard eating might run something like this: the breakfast I described in item 1; for lunch a huge salad made out of Boston lettuce, a whole can of tunafish, slices of cheese, walnuts, carrots, half a can of baby shrimp, and black olives, with an oil, vinegar, lemon, and basil dressing; for dinner, as much rare lamb as you can eat, a casserole of zucchini, tomato, and cheese, wild rice with fresh morels, and a bottle of Chateau Timberlay.

But let's say you don't want to eat like that all the time. That you get cravings for pizza, spaghetti, mashed potatoes —softish, high-carb things. Then do this: Monday through Wednesday eat strictly hard; on Thursday eat a *little* soft, maybe one meal; Friday and Saturday eat very hard again; and on Sunday, pig out—eat everything soft you have wanted all week. I call this the "Three and One, Two and One Hard-Soft Eating Schedule," and it really works. Next to eating hard all the time—and there are very few of us who can do that—it is the best way to eat for staying hard.

11. I happen to believe that bourbon is harder than scotch, and that gin (made from a berry) is harder than vodka (made from potatoes); but I have no scientific evidence. I *know* that good wine is harder than good beer; and that both wine and beer if they are less than good are soft.

12. Try to eat dinner at least two hours before you go to bed and to eat nothing after that. Drinking anything but cognac or Calvados after dinner is soft.

And finally, be sure to chew your food—it is soft not to.